LOOK, I SHRUNK GRANDMA

A Psychiatrist's Guide to Nursing Homes, Dementia, and End of Life

Karen Severson M.D.

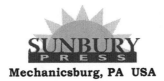

Mechanicsburg, PA USA

Published by Sunbury Press, Inc.
Mechanicsburg, Pennsylvania

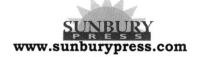

www.sunburypress.com

Copyright © 2018 by Karen Severson, M.D.
Cover Copyright © 2018 by Sunbury Press, Inc.

Sunbury Press supports copyright. Copyright fuels creativity, encourages diverse voices, promotes free speech, and creates a vibrant culture. Thank you for buying an authorized edition of this book and for complying with copyright laws by not reproducing, scanning, or distributing any part of it in any form without permission. You are supporting writers and allowing Sunbury Press to continue to publish books for every reader. For information contact Sunbury Press, Inc., Subsidiary Rights Dept., PO Box 548, Boiling Springs, PA 17007 USA or legal@sunburypress.com.

For information about special discounts for bulk purchases, please contact Sunbury Press Orders Dept. at (855) 338-8359 or orders@sunburypress.com.

To request one of our authors for speaking engagements or book signings, please contact Sunbury Press Publicity Dept. at publicity@sunburypress.com.

ISBN: 978-1-62006-752-9 (Trade paperback)
ISBN: 978-1-62006-753-6 (Mobipocket)

Library of Congress Control Number: 2018930094

FIRST SUNBURY PRESS EDITION: January 2018

Product of the United States of America
0 1 1 2 3 5 8 13 21 34 55

Set in Bookman Old Style
Designed by Crystal Devine
Cover by Lawrence Knorr
Edited by Lawrence Knorr

Continue the Enlightenment!

Dedication

I WROTE THIS BOOK after spending years watching human suffering and feeling helpless at times to stop it. My book is dedicated to those suffering from this horrible illness called dementia. It was written with the hope I could give voice to those who no longer have a voice as this disease destroys their words. They are my teachers to whom I owe a great deal. If I can stop just a small part of their suffering by helping others to understand the illness from my viewpoint, then all my efforts will not be in vain. It is also dedicated to those people who believe in you when you do not believe in yourself—Mailyn Paredes (my wife), Renee Clark Esq., Terry Biemer P.A., Larry Melby, Ellen Brown R.N, and one of my special residents Judith Price. Judith is a fighter and someone I greatly admire. I owe profound thanks to all the nursing home staff who struggle with the same issues as I do and allow me to vent—Shelly, Dierdre, Carol, Paula, MoNica, Laurie, and Kate Quinn. Lastly, there is my editor Helen Myers, who is as smart as she is funny. She helped me not to quit each time I told her I was ready to stop. She pushed me to put all my ideas down, and as I say to my three children, "always do the best you can."

Contents

CHAPTER 1

Let the Shrinking Begin

> ➤ Finally, a tell-all book from a doctor who works at the heart of this situation.
> ➤ It is important to help Grandma. She is a "love nugget."
> ➤ The importance of perspective and humor when dealing with dementia, death, and dying.
> ➤ The QQ equation: Quantity versus Quality.

"Do They Think I'm Crazy?"

It's time for a psychiatrist to do a "tell-all" book on nursing homes, dementia, and your grandmother. Yes, grandma needs shrinking, and I am more than willing to do it. I've seen thousands of elderly in nursing homes at this point. I have been up and down every urine-decorated hallway and food-splattered dining room. I am actually pretty tired, but not giving up. I am ready for the next customer. The next customer could be your mother.

You never know how that first minute will go with a new elderly patient until you walk into the room. I wish I could record the look on some of their faces when they realize I have been asked to evaluate them. No one ever tells them that I am coming. "Why do they think I need you? Do they think I am crazy?" is the usual response. I have developed several appropriate answers to that question, one being, "I hear you are crazy and I came to see with my own eyes." No! Of course I don't say that! I say, "Is it true what they said about you?"

Okay, I will be serious (which I find completely boring). I always do the mature thing and educate them that we really don't use the "crazy" word any longer. I may tell them "I consider crazy running down the halls naked, and as you clearly have clothes on, all is good." I know, it's a broad definition of crazy, but it always makes them laugh and it gets me in the door.

I realized very quickly that people are afraid of psychiatrists in general and even more so in their grandmother's bedroom. I thought we were not worse than the dentist, but I think we are—somewhere in between a toe clipping and tooth pulling in order of avoidance. I have had families ask me, "What's the point in seeing a psychiatrist?" Yes, it is hard not to feel totally useless at that point.

Helping Grandma

Grandma is old, but she is not beyond helping. Age doesn't always make you set in your ways. Well, time does seem to settle things, but it does not always cement things. I saw in a feel-good magazine once how a ninety-year-old woman stated she always wished she would be learning till the end of her life. She would appreciate a good shrink. What an awesome attitude. I hope I end up feeling the same way too at her age. Although there are days I think, this woman needs to take a break from time to time. Doesn't she get tired?

Oh my friend, there is so much to tell. I want to take you into the world of nurses and doctors, what they say and think. Yes, you all see the nurses and aides staring back at you from the nurses' station when you walk in the home. Many times they stare at me too. Sometimes maybe they just have gas—who knows. Maybe, it is something deeper. You don't really know what the staff in nursing homes are thinking. Well, I am going to take a stab at interpreting for you what they might be thinking. It may be good, possibly bad, or it may be as useless as adding gravy to the nursing home mystery meat to make it taste better. How do I know all this? I have worked in nursing homes day in and day out for the last twenty years. I see the sick and dying to the wild and rowdy. I have always struggled on how to refer to them. They all hate the words "geriatric," "senior," "elderly," blah blah blah. There is no perfect word, but I like to think of them as my love nuggets. Why nuggets? Well, we do shrink as we age, hence the "nugget" factor. They are little nuggets of love. I can't lie, there are some mean nuggets too—but most I love. This book is for and about my love nuggets.

Now for the serious side. It's so hard to be serious in this world. If you see and take everything seriously, you'll burn out fast. Actually, I did burn out eventually, but I think I squeaked out a few more years with being able to laugh. Humor is one of the highest coping skills we can develop. Laughing at ourselves and others must happen. Even in death and dying I can find humor. Don't worry; it takes a while to get there on that one. Once you get over the initial shock of all these life and death subjects, it is easier to laugh. We watch as people become ill, suffer in pain, or die. You have to admit, it's hard to cope with it all. Even the subject of dying: it doesn't seem like a laughing matter. Trust me, I will find a way to the humor in just about any situation. Apparently this is how my brain works; I just decided to accept it. It will take a while for you to get there, to discover the light and humorous side of a difficult situation, so sit back and enjoy the ride.

There are several other issues we have to cover. Life in the nursing home, what is it really like? I have the behind-the-scenes undercover view. I have been in all kinds of homes. Rich ones, poor ones, good ones, and really smelly ones. By the way, the sniff test is not always the best indicator of good and bad homes. It might just mean the builders chose carpet not realizing people would be urinating in the air conditioning units and in decorative trees in the corners. Carpets sure hold smell. I offer a chapter about how to pick a home; I have done this work so long, I wanted to offer my advice.

However, this book is focused on exploring dementia and what its like for love nuggets with dementia to be in homes. If you think about it, we get to leave, and the residents have to stay all night. I know, you feel guilty. I wish I could help you on that one. I think they have books on dealing with guilt. But I can actually make you feel even worse. Not only do the residents have to stay, but they also have to deal with brain and body issues on top of it. I know, you would not be reading this book unless you did have some degree of guilt.

Making the "Right" Decisions

All kidding aside, I'm not trying to make it worse. I just want to explain what dementia really looks like and issues that arise with dementia. I think in the end, it will actually help your guilt. I know what you are dealing with—you will hopefully be a pro and make the best decisions for your family. There really are no "right" decisions, there are only well thought-out ones. It's weighing all the facts and coming to what is best for your parent. It will sometimes be for situations that seem impossible, probably because they *are* impossible. You just have to make some sort of decision and go with it. Get used to the guilt and learn to ignore it as much as possible.

Another way I deal with guilt is by trying to build up good karma. I figure I may end up as a nursing home resident one day. I get asked that repeatedly by my patients, "Wouldn't you be depressed if you were here?" Here is how I would love to answer that question in my head. My thought is that if I am going into a home, I am going to go out with a bang. I want at least one food fight. I will look for a gay nursing home as well, since gay men do the best decorating and party planning. I am also hoping they will legalize marijuana in nursing homes. I will look for a home called Woodstock Nursing and Rehab. I one day may actually say this to someone to just see their reaction. I am hoping most would want to sign up. I would remind them to hook up with a crafty family member who can sneak scotch into your bedside Styrofoam cup. Plenty of homes have bars, but trying to get much alcohol with the eight to ten other medications, you have to take is not so easy.

The QQ Equation

You would think I was a total addict and partier, but I am actually not. I just believe in what I call "the QQ equation." This equation is just something I invented to help me make decisions about life in a home. It actually is the *quality* of a life versus *quantity* of life, hence the QQ equation. Let me give you an example of what I mean by this equation in a scenario that comes up frequently. I have seen diabetics who love chocolate. So say this diabetic keeps eating chocolate and then develops poorly controlled diabetes. Should they stop eating chocolate? Your gut response is: "of course!" Your diabetic may lose their eyesight or kidneys if they don't control their sugars. Now what if they have lost a foot to the disease or a kidney because they have been ill for some time. So at this point, do you avoid all foods that give you pleasure if your quality of life is suffering? What if I am that same diabetic with horrible heart, kidney, or circulation issues? Does the situation change for you? Maybe you need to hand over that chocolate nice and slow? I personally, at that point, would just go for the Oreos. I don't want to know I have an expected short *quantity* of life and avoid anything that gives me some *quality*. Others may see the solution differently, but again there are no "right" answers. This is just one small example of hundreds of decisions we have to make on daily basis. I like to use my QQ equation as one factor to consider.

I do run into opposition when I try to apply the QQ equation. There is sometimes a price a resident pays for going for quality of life over quantity. Let me explain. I get all kinds of requests to see "noncompliant" residents. No nursing home wants a person who can't follow the rules. If you don't follow the rules, the home gets in trouble. The state surveyors are looking at every decision made and the consequences of those decisions. The diabetic with the high blood sugars makes it look like nurses are not doing their jobs. The complications of the diabetes make it look even worse. What if the patient develops a foot ulcer or pressure sore from the poorly controlled diabetes? You now have a wound care issue. The state surveyors, who visit on a regular basis, look at wounds closely. Surveyors finding wounds can ruin the home's reputation and open doors to the lawyers. The Oreo cookie is becoming less and less appealing for the facility. I get called in to make that person "behave" and follow the diet. Of course, families are also not happy when a non-compliant resident develops complications. I would not expect them to be! Sadly, there is not a perfect way to make a resident be compliant! We can't hide every cookie in the building. Trust me, I have seen diabetics wipe out cookie trays. As you can see, there are always constant issues that have to be weighed and reweighed. The decisions for me always go back to what improves the *quality* of life, regardless of whom it upsets. The resident determines what is the *quality* of life they seek. Each decision a patient or family makes is very interconnected to a number of other issues—whether it is obvious or not. I think this is why I made the QQ equation. It helps lead to solutions in some horrible situations.

In the next chapter, I'll tell you a bit of my personal story. You may find in it parallels to your own life.

CHAPTER 2

My Personal Journey: Exposure to Dying

➤ Facing mortality.
➤ Mom's troubled life.
➤ Childhood with my mother.
➤ Mom's cancer—waiting for a cure from God.
➤ Frank honest talk with a dying parent.
➤ Letting go.

Before I go on to talk about nursing homes and dementia in a deeper degree, I want to tell you a story about me. If you know my story, you will see how I have formed the opinions that lead me to where I am today. But first a quote to get you in that mental space:

> Everything that is born from causes and conditions is perishable. Impermanence contradicts our feelings of the lasting quality of time and our human desire for immortality. It is the unbearable for the ordinary beings that have not trained their mind to conceive of the world's absence of reality. Denial of impermanence represents one of the main causes of suffering in our existence.
> —*His Holiness, the Dalai Lama*

Oh! I said I would start slowly. Oops! Well that quote is about as serious as a punch in the gut. The denial of death. But he is right, we need to think about these issues, so let me begin softly and slowly to take you there. This is your second warning in case you want to back out now.

Mom

My story is where all our stories begin—with our mothers—the first relationship we form and, to me, the deepest. She is also the person with whom I first experienced what death was like.

Mom passed away many years ago, but her life taught me so much about death and illness. She died of breast cancer while I was a medical student. Of course, as a doctor, I wanted to use what she taught me for my patients. I don't know if she ever knew I was watching her so closely.

My mother was a real firecracker, always outgoing, and she loved to say things to startle people. She used to smoke a cigar for the shock and awe effect. Back then,women just never did these things. I think her personality reminds me of the many elderly I see now; anything they think of will come out of their mouths—for better or worse. She was a beautiful Italian woman, with voluptuous lips and high cheekbones. She was a natural beauty, and she looked very Sophia Loren. She had had a few modeling stints, but she threw away all the pictures. She never really appreciated her own beauty. As with many models, her self-image was horrible. She was emotionally needy and reliant on others to prop her up and boost her self-image.

She had a horrible upbringing, and later she married to find love. She had three children but abandoned them to foster care. She was not emotionally available for them, and she was so wounded. After meeting my father, he did help her get back two of the three children. The third, no one heard from again. That very sadness of losing her son tore at her soul to no end. She would tell us it was her biggest regret.

My Childhood: The Deer Head on the Wall

I was born in her second batch of kids, the middle child. I always saw her sadness even when I was very young. I intuitively knew she had us to help give her the love she so desperately needed. I was that shy and introspective kid. I observed everything, even when no one knew I was looking. I watched what made her happy and what made her sad. I tried to make sure she had more of the stuff that made her happy. She thought of me as most like her. I had her high cheekbones and big smile, a smile that felt like it took up most of my face. I was her mini me. My siblings were not happy about my status. They did not know that it came at a high price.

My real dilemma started when I was about sixteen, when she developed breast cancer. I had no idea what was really going on, as no one would explain it to us kids. She came home one day with a large surgical incision, and her breast was gone. I honestly had no clue what that was about. I just felt a little queasy looking at it. So as you can see, obviously my family did not discuss feelings a great deal. It was like when you walk into some home and see a dead deer head on the wall. You want to say, "What the hell is that god awful thing," but you have to keep your mouth shut so as not to offend anyone. The deer's head stares right at you and you feel completely uncomfortable. Okay, let's just look away and try to avoid it. That was what her cancer was like to my family, the big dead deer's head in the room.

She was cancer free for some time. It did return in about five years. She had waited too long to get it treated in the first place. I later asked my father why she didn't try harder to treat it earlier. My father told me she kept waiting for God to heal her. Hmm ... waiting for God to heal her. Figures my Mom tried that—conventional was never her.

Later on in life, I remember reading a story that reminded me of this situation. It was about a man who asked God for help heal his serious illness. His wife sent him several doctors to see if he could be cured. He refused to see the doctors. He was sure God would help. He ended up dying and going to heaven. When he arrived there, he asked God why he had not saved him. God said, "I sent you several doctors to help you but you told them no." I realized then that God sends to you what you need: it's up to you not only to see but to be open to the help or accept it. Well, I guess I could be angry with my mother for just waiting for God to heal her. There were times my heart ached with why she waited for a holy cure. I know how much God meant to her, and this was her chosen path. This was her destiny—the way it was supposed to go. People have to learn things how they need to learn them, not how we think they need to learn. I always knew things happened the way they were supposed to, and I am at peace with that now.

After the surgery, she did finally try a combination of both medical and natural treatments. She had a very quiet oncologist. (I think all oncologists are quiet. I have never met a loud, boisterous one ever.) He did try chemotherapy and radiation on her, but honestly, it was a horrible experience. When you are trying to kill cancer cells, you kill many other cells—that you kind of need. It's like taking a machine gun and blowing apart an ant on the ground. I am not an expert in the field of oncology, but this is just what I learned from my experience with my mother.

Petty Theft and Personal Freedom

Her first natural treatment was in Tijuana, Mexico. As our only vacations were camping in the woods, I imagined that Tijuana was a beautiful resort city. I want to thank my mother now for ruining all foreign travel for me forever after seeing Tijuana. I was scared out of my mind driving through the city. Thank God I was ignorant at that point that I could have been mugged. Yes, we drove through these really scary streets to a medical clinic in name only. They introduced an actually very strange theory of treatment to us. We were told that people with cancer had too much yeast in their bodies. The idea apparently was that yeast lowers your immune system and allows cancer to grow. They, of course, felt both my sister and I were infected with yeast as well. We were encouraged to follow this diet change. It took me a minute to process not eating anything with yeast. I can tell you now with no hesitation, no one stops this girl from eating pizza! I was pretty annoyed at the treatment and knew it was a terrible way to take advantage of a dying person. Of course, she stuck with the diet, which included a strange black liquid they sold her. I still have a leftover bottle in my garage. I keep it as reminder of how someone took advantage of her vulnerability to make money. And then there are my sarcastic times when I wish it was really Jaegermeister. I could invite my friends over for shots. Sadly, I think Jaegermeister might have been more effective for my mother.

On our way back from the clinic to California, we stopped at a souvenir store where I recall one of the more profound moments in my life. I'll never forget it. She was so happy to be there and to actually be traveling. I loved to see it in her eyes. I watched her browse through the store, never recalling she was ill. The next moment I saw her walking away from the store swinging a colorful wind chime in her hand. She looked so free and happy. It was so nice as I had not seen this look in her eye for so long. My sister and I then realized why she was dancing and acting so happy. She was trying to act like nothing was wrong as she was walking out of the store after stealing the ornament. Well, of course I was shocked, but it was mixed with an odd bit of joy. I felt so much freedom in her at that moment. The woman who didn't care about what the world thought of her—that sense of freedom from all of life's restrictions on her face. I wanted this so much for her all the time. Even though stealing is wrong, it gave her a moment of freedom from her inner pain. She laughed at her own momentary insanity to give me a valuable lifelong memory. This made the trip to Mexico completely worth it. Oh yes, we kept that dumb-looking chime.

She did make another trip to Europe without me. She was trying to cure the massive lymphedema in her left arm. The radiation and surgeries prevented her arm from draining fluid, and it swelled three times the normal size. It became very heavy and looked awkward on her thinning body. She wanted it amputated at one point, but the doctors told her this was too risky. What does one do when one runs out of all options? Do you continue to fight and develop more disability, or do you stop and try to enjoy each moment left? How hard it is to stop fighting and just value each and every moment you have with your loved ones? It always affected me deeply that she would have amputated her limb to have relief from pain. What horrible decisions to consider in relief of suffering.

Sharing and Caring at the End: Questions, Questions, Questions

Recently, a daughter visiting in one of my nursing homes brought me back to those feelings. The daughter was with her dying mother. The daughter told me her mother was someone who never really talked about her feelings. She had the "dead-deer-head-in-the-room" syndrome. The mother did have one big very obvious emotion. She was very angry. Her mother was asking her why she didn't just let her die and was quite angry, as she had no quality of life after several strokes.

The daughter couldn't let go. She wanted more medical intervention, which obviously upset her mother more. I just asked the daughter to not make the life or death decisions *that* day. Don't even talk about those things for a moment, I advised her. Instead, I suggested that she just get to know her mother before she died. Her response was that her mother never discussed her feelings. I told her just to ask questions. Ask her as many questions about her life as she could think of before she lost her. Ask her how she knew she fell in love with your father? Did she have any unrealized dreams? What did she really want to be when she grew up? One of those questions might open a previously emotionally closed door. You may connect and understand each other at a level you never knew possible. You may open that door that allows you both to let go of trying to fix or save each other. Just being. My family wasted all that time obsessing about a cure that we missed out on more valuable experiences. I can't get that time back, but she, the daughter visiting my nursing home, could. The relationship she and her mother had might transform out of anger, and then understanding might come.

Even better I suggest, don't wait until someone is ill before you ask these questions.

Final Hours with Mom

So what happened to my mother? Which way did she turn after her cure was hopeless? It's fine to say hopeless. It didn't make her a failure—not in the least. She finally did the best treatment of all: she turned to her feelings. She found a book called *Love Medicine and Miracles* by Dr. Bernie Siegel. He was a surgeon in New Haven, and he actually performed some surgeries on her. Finally, we hit pay dirt—a doctor who was integrating spirit and body. I remember a happy bald man approaching me and shaking my hand. I was surprised to meet a surgeon who was happy and not a white coat with a cocky attitude. He knew I was going to be a doctor and told me I just needed to learn a new language to become a doctor. He made it sound easy. I guess that meant I needed to learn medical terminology,and I would qualify. He probably should have said you would have *no* life for several years while your friends party like rock stars. I think that would have made more sense to me. I actually really loved his book; it had a lot of interesting pictures. I have some ADHD, and any book with a lot of pictures I find awesome. All kidding aside, it mainly had art therapy pictures as he commonly used them in his practice. It allowed patients to tap into emotions they were otherwise unable to discuss. Patients drew their illness and the treatment they were receiving. If patients drew positive pictures about their treatment, he felt they would do better with the cancer.

My mother had her art therapy picture published in the *Hartford Courant* through Dr. Siegel. I was proud. It was a picture of a bright yellow field and a tree stump growing in the lower corner. From the tree was growing a small sprout. The doctor told her the tree represented her life, which had been cut off early from a childhood trauma. She had suffered horrible childhood abuse, both sexually and emotionally. She had rickets from pure neglect as a baby. The small tree sprout in the art therapy picture represented her spirit. It had been cut off from growing after she was traumatized. It finally started re-growing after all these years. It took a horrible cancer for her to start really dealing with the pain of her childhood. In the upper corner there were three birds that represented her three children that she had with my father. She was worried how her cancer and death would affect us. She didn't want to leave us. We were there in the picture as a concern for her. She really was trying to survive for us.

My mother finally died at my medical school. She was on a morphine pump, sleeping deeply. We all had taken pillows off the couches to sleep on the floors around her. They say that people's spirits pass in the wee hours of the morning. They do not want us to see them go. The nurse shook me awake at around 2 a.m., and I looked at her body briefly. I knew she was no longer there in her body, so I did not stay. I stood outside on that cold night staring at the flags on the hospital roof. I imagined her spirit flying away through them. She was finally free.

She fought terribly hard and did suffer at times. Once you live that experience with your parent and then with multiple patients, you do change. You see death very differently. After my mother passed, I starting asking more people about how they felt about death. It was hard to do at times because families can become very upset if you bring up dying. I would do it in private. The patients themselves never seemed upset by my asking. It was as if these patients enjoyed the chance to finally say what they were feeling. People think that if you ask about dying, then somehow you open up the desire for someone to want to die. This is *not* true. People also have the same fear if you ask about suicide. I was also taught in school that asking about suicidal thoughts didn't make people suicidal. Trust me, the more you ask people about dying, the easier it gets. I know this sounds strange, but it can be a very normal conversation. I love to ask people in their nineties the most about death and dying.

I actually had one woman who was so happy she was going to die. The children asked me to see her to decide if she was "handling" her cancer diagnosis appropriately. I felt like I had to give antidepressants to the children, as they were more depressed than she was about her cancer. So you wonder how someone could be happy to die? Well this woman had died once already, and she loved it. She said it was so great she was very unhappy she came back. When she developed cancer years after that experience, she had found her chance to go back and was totally fine with it. I was glad she was able to somehow get rid of all the mother's guilt of leaving her children. She felt she had given her children the wings to fly on their own now. Her gift was immortal. She had served her purpose in life and she was ready.

A Purpose in Life

Just remember, one's purpose in life *is not always seen while you are alive in this world.* Your purpose may be there to teach others lessons in life they need to have to grow. I really believe a death can teach so much about life. I know that may not explain why people have to die, both young and old, but I believe it to be true. I feel one of my mother's purposes in life was to teach me about really living before you die. My purpose is to carry that on so her death was not in vain.

CHAPTER 3

What Is Dementia?

➤ Geriatric psychiatry.
➤ Dementia has no cure.
➤ Neurocognitive disorder.
➤ Doctor–family–patient relationships.
➤ Forms of dementia: Alzheimer's, vascular dementia, Parkinson's disease, Huntington's disease.
➤ Diagnosing vascular dementia.
➤ Aphasia.
➤ Disorientation.
➤ Damage to the frontal lobe.
➤ Dementia and driving.

Making Personal Choices

Despite the stress of my mother's death, I continued on with my medical education for one simple reason. Damn, I had a ton of debt! How else was I going to pay it off!? I made the decision to go into geriatric psychiatry. I have been asked several times why I chose this specialization, as most people find it depressing. Well the answer is threefold. I enjoyed psychiatry as it has a new and different presentation with each patient. I found general medicine boring, as it seemed to be the same old bladder infection, cold, or allergy. I loved neurology, but it was hard to find a neurologic illness with a cure. I wanted something I could cure. I thought that geriatric psychiatry would be a nice combination of general medicine, psychiatry, and neurology. I was actually correct on the issues. It was a good fit for me. I also always loved older people, so it all made sense. Of course, I was working in Florida, the nugget capitol of the United States, and knew I would always have a job. It seemed like a really smart idea.

"Senior Moments"

Let me give you an example of how geriatric psychiatry is a combination of all three—general medicine, psychiatry, and neurology. It's called dementia. Each person has a totally different personality, so a case of dementia is always new and different. It has some medical issues that come up, and it is a neurologic illness. It does not have a cure, but there are things we can do to make it better. I have to admit, it took me a long time to figure dementia out. I could read all the books in the world, but it did not really click for me in the beginning. Geriatric psychiatry involves a great deal of dementia, so I had to get it right. I also realized that people were afraid to discuss dementia or even let me test for it.

I had this brilliant idea one day of running a screening clinic for memory problems at an assisted living facility where I worked. No one showed up! Who really wants to find out they have dementia? I honestly don't blame them—I probably wouldn't want to know either. I felt like an idiot that day and struggled to figure out how we could get patients diagnosed faster. In dementia cases, early intervention is so important for planning. So, if the elderly do not want to know whether they have dementia, then I can write this book to teach families how to recognize it! If you can go through a problem, you can go around it. I am going to teach you all what I have learned—the tricks of the trade.

Tests for Dementia

I will give you my best description of dementia as possible in layman's terms. The only other thing you need to do before I go on is to read the whole chapter before you try to guess at a diagnosis for Grandma. Keep a clear and open mind. Why do I say this? Because it's so hard for us to be objective about our own parents and loved ones. It's so easy to make excuses for those "senior moments." I am sure I would be the same way, as I couldn't even accept my own mother's death until she had twenty-four-hour hospice care. There were also times I just didn't want to believe someone could have dementia, and I was not even related to them. "Oh no please, not this person, they are too stinking awesome to have dementia,"

I would think. I don't want anyone to have dementia, but I have been tempted to give a few super cutie pies a few more clues on my tests so they would score higher points. I could have totally just cheated for them. My heart would start to drop as they were giving wrong answers. There were times I didn't even want to do the tests: avoidance was easier. Unfortunately, I have performed the dementia tests (specifically the Mini Mental Status Exam) so many hundreds of times and have met thousands with the illness, that I can recognize dementia without the tests. It was getting too hard to hide this ability. Dementia was becoming more obvious to me by just listening to how people expressed themselves and processed information, as well as the obvious memory gaps!

Reaction of the Family

The other difficult part for me was the dread of knowing I had to tell someone I thought they had dementia. Even harder—having to tell their spouse or children. I was creamed a few times by families not yet ready to hear such a diagnosis. Because there are no blood tests for dementia, it is easier for people to argue with the diagnosis. I would hear things like, "She just woke up, even I can't remember things when I just wake up." "You don't know what you are talking about; you can't diagnose dementia after one visit." There have been multiple times I have asked families to leave the room while I test because they start answering the questions for Mom. I have to remind them that I am not testing their memory; I am testing their mother's. I had one patient failing the test, and the daughter said to me, "Mom is lying to you. She knows the answer but will not say." It is always a tough decision I have to make: whether the family stays in the room or goes in the hall for a minute as I test memory. If I think it will help with educating the family, and they can avoid answering the questions themselves, please stay. If they are going to argue with me on the standard questions we ask everyone, they have to step out or I can't get a good test. Nothing personal. I wish diagnosis were not this way! It's so hard. It was getting to the point where I would ask the nurses how open the family would be to the diagnosis. Yes, this is one of the things the staff discusses behind the desk—how does the family handle bad news. If I knew a family was easily upset, I would have to weigh keeping my mouth shut. Oh trust me, it was so tempting to put my head in the sand. I have seen other doctors avoid mentioning a diagnosis of dementia, and families loved those doctors. Did I want to be a popular doctor, or did I want to be the doctor who told the truth, despite the consequences. I generally told families the truth. I practiced tons of different ways to break the news of my opinions—so hard to do. If a family were not accepting, I would just mention my concern about the memory issues and tell them to, "just keep an eye on it." At least I tried and did not avoid. Early in my career, I was horrible at taking the anger people would show just hearing my concerns. I suppose by belittling me and my opinions, it is easier for families to avoid facing reality. Either way, it would have helped me to have a book like this to lay the groundwork for such discussions. It just takes so long to explain dementia to loved ones; I felt I was not doing a very good job in the short time available. I see this book as a chance to help other medical workers as well as families struggling with this same issue. I have spoken to many doctors who have also expressed the frustration with the lack of time to explain the illness. Don't get me wrong. Not all families handle a dementia diagnosis poorly. Some are very appreciative that they finally understand why grandma has a totally different personality than before. I just want patients and their loved ones to recognize how hard a struggle it is for medical personnel to discuss the issue with you. It may help smooth over the stress in these tough conversations.

"I have WHAT? Neurocognitive disorder?"

Dementia is so upsetting for people to contemplate that we are even changing the name of the illness. We no longer say "dementia"; we have to say "neurocognitive disorder." It sounds softer and less threatening. I have to say that it will be hard for me to make this change. I can just imagine people saying, "I have what? Neurocognitive disorder?" And I have to answer, "Yes, that is the same as dementia." I feel we just added a whole new step in explanation. Supposedly, part of the reason for the name change is that neurocognitive disorder sounds less frightening for families and patients. I will let you be the judge.

I am going to stick with the old fashioned word for now, "dementia." The most frequent question I am asked is, "Is dementia the same as Alzheimer's?" Yes, it is—about 60 percent of dementia is Alzheimer's and another 30 percent is called vascular dementia. The remainder is a multitude of other dementias that coincide with other illnesses, such as Parkinson's disease or Huntington's disease. All in all, the end results and the treatments are pretty similar. They are all progressive terminal illnesses. Sadly, there really are no cures for these diseases. There are medications that MAY slow the illnesses, but no cures as of yet. I try not to obsess too much on the type of dementia for this reason. If it changed the treatment to know the type of dementia, I would be all over it.

Diabetes and Dementia

I mentioned diabetes when discussing my QQ equation. Diabetes haunts me, as it is a disease where we can possibly prevent dementia. This is why I get so upset at young people not taking care of their health. For example, I just met a really young woman who came to me for treatment of her depression. She wanted me to fill her diabetic medications, as she had let them run out for a few weeks. I couldn't help but be frustrated with her, as I knew what happens when you don't control diabetes. You can develop vascular dementia. If I really wanted to scare her, I knew I could. I could have told her how I knew someone who went blind, or the plethora of people I knew with foot and leg amputations. Diabetes causes all kinds of destruction to the old noggin. Well, I did try to scare her. She looked pretty mad at me at the moment. It was one of the few times when the "scare technique" actually worked. She was on top of all her medications and blood sugars by the next visit. They say sometimes you are not helping people unless they are angry with you—this was totally true for this woman.

Vascular Dementia

Let us explain this vascular dementia in greater detail. It is related not only to diabetes, but high blood pressure and high cholesterol as well. I like to use analogies when I explain vascular dementia. Vascular is another word for the vessels carrying blood throughout the body. I refer to the blood vessels as pipes similar to the plumbing in a house. Diabetes, like high blood pressure and high cholesterol, destroys your pipes. As the blood is being pumped, the pipes the blood passes through become progressively smaller and smaller. The tiniest of tiny of these pipes are easily damaged by the high blood pressure banging on their walls. Bad cholesterol seeps into the walls of the pipes and grows like stalagmites in a cave. High blood sugars harden the arteries like that glaze over crème brûlée. I had fun creating these analogies, and I hope they create a clear image of what's happening in your body. Let's add a few more interesting analogies: the flushing toilet analogy. Imagine the pipes flowing from your toilet being almost completely clogged. You flush it that one more time, and a little piece of toilet paper hits that mother load. We have all been there, running for the plunger with our pants down. I feel it's a good description of that little blood clot (the toilet paper) finally hitting your arteries clogged with cholesterol. These tiny millimeter-sized pipes clog and stop the blood from flowing to parts of your brain. A brain starved of blood results in a stroke. The brain tissue dies, and the stroke patient develops a weak arm or a drooping face. Sometimes, the doctor may not see any obvious neurological deficits. We call these silent strokes. Over the years, these tiny silent strokes can accumulate. What the family may start to notice instead of the drooping face, are short-term memory complaints. If you look at the CT scans of these patients, there are multiple tiny spots scattered throughout the scan. Isn't it just like doctors to refer to everything as spots? But, this is what they look like! It looks like your brain was shot with spitballs that land randomly. These spots are actually what are described as "microvascular changes" or "lacunar infarcts." They are the hallmark of vascular dementia.

One other clue that helps the doctor tell if it is vascular versus Alzheimer's dementia is what we call "stepwise declines." Vascular dementia has a stepwise decline-type presentation. For instance, one day your mother is completely normal. The next minute she is acting completely confused and not processing information. You run to the emergency room, and the doctor tells you the CT scan is normal. You know you are not imagining her confusion, as she is different from yesterday. The hospital must have missed something! Well, most likely the damage was so small that it was not showing up on the scans. I have seen many families so confused by this. "They told me all the tests are negative," they say. I let families know it was probably a small stroke that could not be picked up on a test. I try to reassure them that the confusion can gradually clear after this event, but Grandma may never return to exactly how she was before. This is the stepwise decline—classic for vascular dementia. The patient drops, levels off, and then drops again. This is why I tell families to find out if the radiologist mentioned microvascular changes or lacunar infarcts in the radiology report, as these are signs of vascular dementia. Most times, the ER doctors will just tell you there are no acute major strokes. You want to know if they have the little damage as well. If the report does mention multiple spots on the CT scan, there is no way to know exactly when the tiny strokes occurred. All one can say is that the mini strokes have happened at some point in time. If there are enough of these baby strokes that accumulate, vascular dementia can result. So in summary, Alzheimer's dementia has a more gradual and progressive decline—a smooth roll down a hill. Vascular dementia presents as much more abrupt decline followed by a period of stability. The other clear difference is that someone with Alzheimer's disease generally will have a completely normal CT scan or, at the most, some possible brain shrinkage.

Alzheimer's Dementia

Let us focus more now on the Alzheimer's dementia. We all really know it by its hallmark symptom of short-term memory loss. I used to have a guy with dementia who told me the same joke over and over. He told me he had CRS, which means, "Can't remember shit." I will never forget that guy—he laughed so hard each time he told the joke. But, he pretty much summarized short-term memory loss in that joke. Of course, many obviously forgetful people argue with me that they can remember everything from their past. They challenge me to quiz them on everything they have ever learned. Of course, this would be impossible, but I have to break it to them that I am more interested in their short-term memory. I just want to ask them if they can remember three words in five minutes. It is a bit of an awkward moment. This type of patient generally wants me to focus on their long-term memory to avoid me noticing their short-term memory loss. If you do have long-term memory issues, then the patient is fairly well along in the illness, and I probably wouldn't need to test them at all as they would most likely have dementia. People with dementia are unable to lay down new memories, like those three words I give them. Sometimes there are the obvious clues that the patient has memory issues anyone can notice without a test. I think we have all met that person who tells the same story over and over as if it were the first time. The memory loss I am discussing is not about forgetting people's names or where you left your keys. This type of forgetfulness is normal. The memory loss with dementia is more pervasive. They forget everything they just heard, not just names.

Aphasia

I think people also confuse normal age-related memory loss with dementia. I don't want to get too deep into details, but dementia requires more than just memory loss to make the diagnosis. We also look for issues with the use of language. Have you ever heard people end sentences and start new ones when they forget the word they wanted to use? "Oh yeah, what's that called?" If you can't recall the word you want to use, the next best thing is to just change the subject. People with dementia will commonly do this subject change so no one will notice they are struggling to find a word. It is a way to cover up what is called "aphasia." It is the inability to name objects or generate words. For example someone with aphasia might say, "Help me find my, uh, that thing you shave your face with." The higher your IQ and education, the better you are at hiding this symptom. This is why it is so hard for me to always diagnose dementia in highly educated people. I am sure aphasia is terribly annoying and extremely frustrating for people. It can start out gradually and progresses to the point that people no longer make sense. I will hear people say, "I am so stupid," when they can't find the word. I remind them that it has nothing to do with intellect; it is a symptom of the illness.

If you are not sure if someone has aphasia, there is a good quick and dirty test I can give you. Tell the person you will give them a letter and then they have to name as many words with that letter as they can in one minute's time. You only tell them the letter after they understand the instructions. They can't use names for people, and they have to name at least eleven words in that minute. Please do not choose letters like "a" or "f" for obvious reasons. I suppose the letter "d" has a few curse words as well. I only had to make this mistake once as this one guy had a field day embarrassing me with inappropriate words. Anyway, the less words you can think of, the more likely you are developing aphasia. And the higher the person's IQ, the longer they can fool you on these tests.

Hey! What day is it?: "Patient is alert and oriented by 3"

Another criteria to make the dementia diagnosis is disorientation. A question I have asked a million times, "Do you know what the date is today?" Oh yes, it annoys me as much as it annoys the person I am asking. I know they have usually been asked already, but I have to do it one more time. Here is what I have learned from this exercise. The more confused person is, the more they argue about having to answer the questions. "Of course I know the date!" Then I reply, "Okay, then just tell me so we can say we did the test." They think that if they get angry at my question, I will give up and move on. Oh no! I am like a dog with a bone. I will ask it several ways if needed. I am happy if they get at least the month and the year correct. The day of the week and the date are hopefully correct within a few days. I love asking the season. Countless times I have thought it would be such an easy question, but apparently it fools many people. Some do not understand what I mean by season. I suppose this is part of the aphasia. I have to eventually name all four seasons and let the patient try to guess between them all. In Florida I suppose we only have two seasons, hot and warm. You would really have to know the month to get the season down here. The next five questions (a total of ten) on orientation are the name of the place, floor of building, city, county, and state. I found out that many people do not even know the name of the county where they are located. I have several times just asked them what county they vote in, and that triggers the memory.

I was reminded about one scary aspect of disorientation the other day. I was walking out of a store when an elderly woman approached me. I was not even at work; how could this be happening? I swear I am a nugget magnet. She was frantic and asked me where Forest Hill Blvd was located. Well, we were on the street she was asking about. She could not find her way home. I felt awful. I was with my small children, and it was hard for me to do much. They were screaming and pulling at my legs. I tried to ask her who I could call for her, and she refused. I re-oriented her and she went on her way, refusing all help. I kept thinking of her children and how they might have no idea what their mother was doing. Maybe they saw mom getting forgetful, but they would probably not antici- pate her getting lost in a familiar area. I suppose they were lucky she walked up to someone who would not try to take advantage of her situation. Someone could have easily tried to take a credit card. This is the scary part of disorientation, people becoming lost or injured. They call it a "Silver Alert" in Florida. All the more reason to get diagnosed for dementia sooner.

I am going to tell you a secret about disorientation. Everyone in the medical field knows this secret, we just never talk about it. Nurses and doctors stink at checking orientation. We hate asking all those same questions. If someone seems "with it," we don't even bother running through all ten questions. Since I am very obses- sive about it, I will run through at least eight orientation questions if I am concerned. I love catching the nurses when they assume a person is all "with it." I say to them, "then why did they tell me it's 1954?" Trust me, some patients can easily fool us all. We need to make sure we catch those people who are early in the illness. We are not helping the situation if we in the medical field write that well repeated phrase, "patient is alert and oriented by 3" (3 means person, place, and time). We can't write that unless we actually do the test.

The Frontal Lobe: "Nice Butt!"

Last, but not least, is the most complicated part of dementia. It is called frontal lobe or executive function. The frontal lobe is the executor of brain, the part of your brain that brings facts, emotions, memories, and logic together to make decisions. If you are old enough to remember *Star Trek*, then you will get it when I say Dr. Spock was the frontal lobe of the Starship Enterprise. He was the guy who was gathering all the information like a computer and spitting out a logical answer. The only way in which he was different from a frontal lobe, was in that he did not allow emotion to factor into his decisions. The frontal lobe also stops you from doing something that would be considered socially inappropriate. This is why we don't burp loudly in front of others. It is also why we do not ask a beautiful woman passing by us for a kiss or say "nice butt." What about that person who cuts in front of you in line? You would slap them silly if not for your frontal lobe.

What if you damage your frontal lobe as with dementia? I think you all probably have been around people with frontal lobe issues without really realizing it. We have all had that visit to gramps and were worried what he would say. Hopefully, the most you would hear is a few choice curse words in front of the kids. The worst is what he plans to do with Grandma later. The same issues happen in nursing homes. There probably is not a nurse alive who has not been spanked on the tush while passing out medications. Several nurses have asked me to help them with that issue. I wish there was a pill for that one! But sorry! The frontal lobe is not putting on the brakes!

I bet now you are wondering what I do for these sexual issues. Well, there is one medication I do have for hypersexual men. But the medication does not work on hypersexual women. I am always shocked when I get that occasional woman who can't keep her hands off the men. I thought we lost our sex drive after menopause. Heck no! Apparently some women have a secret power pack of testosterone. I thought men would not mind this type of woman around either. Totally wrong. I had this one woman chasing all the male packages in the home. She was never tired. The men were running from her. There was nothing I could do! Finally, I recommended they move her to an all female unit. Just so you know, this hypersexual behavior is a sign of frontal lobe impairment. It is not a sign that your loved one has suddenly wanted to get back into the dating pool.

Aggression

There is darker side to frontal lobe injuries from dementia—aggression. Aggression is actually a very serious issue, as well as the most common symptom I treat. Again, people are not neurologically able to inhibit that burst of anger they feel. I have seen people get kicked, punched, tripped, and even bit. I recall watching an eighty-five-year-old woman, who weighed probably 90 lbs., try to trip another woman. I was also punched really hard in the arm once. A woman was trying to elope from a home, and I was in between her and freedom. I was a cocky young athlete, thinking what can she possibly do to me? I am pretty sure that any person alive, at any age, can do some damage with a little boost of adrenaline. Let's just say she humbled me. All kidding aside, aggression is very scary. The worst I have personally seen is an aide loose the tip of her finger in a door. Apparently, the woman with dementia did not want this aide in her room. She decided to slam the door on her. When the aide held up her hand, her finger was caught in the door and the finger was severed. I am sad to say, it was crushed so badly that they were unable to sew the finger chunk back on.

Seeing these types of injures makes you much more paranoid each time you see a new resident with the aggression issue. You can't predict which person will really hurt someone. You have to assume anyone could do damage, even if they were the sweetest person in the world in their younger days. Another one of my aides was punched so hard in the abdomen that she was sent to the emergency room. The ER called asking if charges were going to be pressed against the man who assaulted her. Apparently, this resident had done some type of damage for them to call back. We can't press charges against a resident with dementia. However, there have been several people living in the nursing home community with dementia who have been arrested for assault. It was common enough experience in Palm Beach that an organization was formed to keep aggressive citizens with dementia out of jail.

Not all aggression is this severe. Most of the time it is just slaps causing bruising. This is why homes try to get pictures of bruises so the families do not blame the staff for the marks. I have also seen plenty of broken hips from one resident pushing down another. It's like a playground of kids pushing each other when they are angry, except these people have osteoporosis. Kids bounce when they fall; the elderly break bones. Children do not finish developing their frontal lobes until their early twenties. This is why teens have trouble stopping risky behaviors.

Screamers: "Kill Me!"

One other similarity between young children and elderly is loud screaming. I mean people with normal lobes scream too, but their frontal lobe gets them to stop eventually. There are times when you walk into a home and hear someone screaming at the top of their lungs. One example is when I used to take my daughter Tori with me to the homes with our pet corgi. We named all our corgis after Christmas reindeer. Cupid loved to go for pet therapy. I was mortified when Tori and Cupid saw this one famous screamer we named Adeline. She would yell, "KILL ME" at the top of her lungs—repeatedly. I looked at Tori in fear that this woman would traumatize her for life. I was relieved when she understood the woman really didn't want us to murder her. She basically just wanted someone to spend time with her. Adeline could actually have somewhat appropriate conversations in between her yelling, "kill me." Several times people would stop and explain to her that they did not feel they could kill her, but if she needed something else they could help. I was often worried about what the visitors touring the building would think. I also felt bad for her peers, who had to listen to her for hours. Clearly, it would be pretty agitating. I actually had a call the other day to see a woman with dementia who was shaking one of the screamers. She just wanted her to stop. I decided to treat the screamer and not the woman who shook her. It made sense. If I had dementia I would consider shaking someone screaming constantly to get them to stop. I am glad my frontal lobe is working, and I don't shake the residents.

The Broken Record!

Adeline is a good example of another frontal lobe issue called perseveration. I think most people will identify this one quickly. It is when someone gets "stuck" on an idea or an issue. It is like the broken record skipping on the same line of a song. Our frontal lobe is supposed to stop our brain from that repetition, but in dementia, all bets are off. For Adeline, she persevered on wanting someone to kill her. Let me provide one more example, I had one resident ask me about fifty times, "when is the bus coming to take us home." The first few times you explain the buses were cancelled for the day. You feel so smart for coming up with that one; they are satisfied with the answer and leave. Five minutes later, they are back asking the same question as they forgot you even had this conversation. They are persevering on the bus. I generally call the nurse at this point and try to get the resident involved in an activity. Typical doctor—call the nurse to save us. Sadly, there are also no medications to stop perseveration, as it is a neurological symptom. I am sure there are many families out there begging for a cure though. It is really stressful for families to have to answer the same question repeatedly.

"It's Not Me, It's You!": Loss of Insight

Last but not least, is "insight." This symptom of dementia is the hardest to explain. Dementia destroys the insight into the fact that you have an illness at all. Many with dementia, not all, feel everyone else has the problem and not them. This is also part of the frontal lobe injury. They do not get why their family wants them to sell the car, stop living alone, or hand over the checkbook. Loss of insight seems more common in Alzheimer's dementia than in vascular dementia. If those tiny strokes only hit the memory or language areas of the brain, then they keep the insight area. They know they are loosing their memories and it really bothers them. People with Alzheimer's may not even notice they have a memory issue at all. They can't understand why people are bothering them. This is a sure sign they are developing dementia, loss of insight into the obvious problem. Loss of insight can lead to other problems. I see more people develop paranoia with loss of insight. For example, how many times have you lost your belongings and feel frustrated by it. You know you were just being absent minded, and you lost it. People with dementia do not feel they lost anything. There is no way it was their fault. It had to be your fault. You, or someone else like the CNA, stole your stuff! There is no convincing them otherwise. Next thing you know, the police are called. I mean things can get stolen in nursing homes, but most likely the missing object rolled under the bed.

"But I never had a ticket!"

Here is a serious example of insight loss—trying to stop people from driving when obviously it is dangerous. I have heard hundreds of times: "I never had a ticket!" Luckily, that is not how we decide whether it is safe for you to drive. Sadly, every now and then we get an older person in our hospital involved in a serious motor vehicle accident. It is devastating, as it could have possibly been prevented. It is so hard to take a car away from someone. They just don't understand the dangers of driving with dementia. I have even had people tell me they would kill themselves if we took their car. I totally understand why they are upset. Again, there are no right decisions, only the best decision. I don't want someone to be harmed, so we are going to have to loosen the spark plugs of the car.

Driving a car also requires multiple parts of the brain, vision, reaction times, good judgment, processing all the information into your brain quickly. The brain must also deal with how to process objects moving in space around you. Cars cutting you off, or stopping suddenly is handled by what is called the visual spatial areas in the brain. I think that if people understood the facts, they would understand why stopping dementia patients from driving is so important. There is actually a bedside test for your visual spatial areas. It is called the clock draw test. It actually tests frontal lobe and visual spatial areas. It can be found online if you want to try the test. You ask someone to draw a circle and then add in all the numbers. You then ask them to set the big and little hands of the clock to 2 p.m. I have seen so many errors on what you would think to be such a simple test. I see people put number one through twelve on only half of the clock. People sometimes ask me to look at a clock to remember how it is done, and still are not able to draw one. They are not able to set the hands to the correct times. A clock draw is testing how your brain "sees" things in space. Can you visualize it in your brain and draw it? It's a rough and dirty way to test the visual spatial centers. If someone fails terribly at the clock, I would not want them to be driving. I do not base my diagnosis entirely on the clock, but it is a large part of it.

Well, we are at the end of the chapter. To summarize, dementia is a brain disease causing changes in memory, language, orientation, frontal lobe function, and insight. I hope this helps even a few of you to apply what many books describe about dementia. I also hope it helps you being open to doctors and nurses when they try to broach the subject. We all have good intentions, and we know how horribly frightening a diagnosis of dementia can be for you. We just want to help you plan and prepare as well as help your loved one deal with the illness. You are becoming their caretaker and need all the weapons you have to fight the stress. Knowledge is a powerful weapon. Fear of the illness only makes all these issues more difficult to deal with, and they drive a wedge between you and the medical field trying to help you. I get afraid as well, but just let the fear pass and keep reaching out. We can all get through this together.

CHAPTER 4

Nursing Home Dilemmas

➤ Relocating to a nursing home.
➤ Medicare and nursing homes.
➤ When to use medication.
➤ The noncompliant resident.
➤ Assisted living facilities.
➤ Wandering.
➤ Patient aggression.
➤ Personal relationships in the nursing home setting.
➤ Paranoia.
➤ Psychosis.
➤ Sundowning.
➤ Depression and delirium.

Now that you have a grasp of dementia, I want to go over a few typical dilemmas we see in nursing homes. I am kept really busy, and there are days I wonder, "Is this really life, or is this a fantasy." No my friend, it's all real. When you close you eyes and shake your head, you are still standing in Tropical Oasis Nursing Home and Rehab. Breathe it in baby, breathe it in. So how does one get a one-way ticket to this hot spot? Well, people are clearly not rushing to get in line.

Many times, it is a pretty sudden decision to relocate. It can happen after someone falls at home and breaks a hip. Most are then sent to a nursing home temporarily for physical therapy. The hospital tells them, "It's just for a short time and then you can go home. You just need to get your strength back." It all sounds good. Hospitals never lie, only nursing homes do. If you sense a little bitterness, you are correct. The hospitals have the glory of saving

29

the person, and the nursing homes get the hard job of dealing with the aftermath. After the arrival at the home, each person will then receive about four to six weeks of therapy on Medicare, and two additional weeks if you decided to buy a managed Medicare policy like Humana. If you succeed physically, you can go home. If you fail physically, or are too confused to live alone, you go to Plan B. The home social workers will then begin scouring your finances to see how you can afford "long term care."

Introducing Grandma to a Nursing Home: "I hate it!" "Forget it!" "No way!" "I disown you!"

So how do you break it to Grandma that she is not leaving? Since no one wants to always come right out and drop that bomb on them, we just keep delaying their discharge over and over. Grandma will keep asking us when she is going home, and we will just as persistently avoid telling her that she can't leave. If they are "with it" and do not have dementia, we obviously can be more upfront. If they have dementia and are unable to process all the reasons they need to stay, then we use the delayed approach. Then the family slowly starts to move in their belongings, and the deal is done. Most are very resistant to the idea understandably. They let staff and the family know, "I hate it," "forget it," "no way," and "I disown you." This is when I am called in. My job is to help them "adjust!" In other words, I also get yelled at for about ten minutes on how horrible we all are for keeping her there.

Adjusting to the Nursing Home Environment

Eventually, many do adjust well. Then there are those who will haunt you until they die. Gramps will remind you every time you see him that he hates what you have done to him. Also, that you do not visit enough. Some patients forget you are visiting them daily, and they accuse you of never visiting. I suppose you can leave a "proof of the visit" somewhere. But basically, you are damned if you do and damned if you don't. As a result, I'm sure many families start to avoid the constant guilt trip even though they do make efforts. Of course, some family members may eventually stop visiting completely, due to the constant harassment and just general guilt. But it is not all gloom and doom, and some residents adjust well after a few months. I am more referring to those who are really shocked and understandably angry they are not allowed to leave.

They are usually the residents with confusion. They tell me, "There is nothing wrong with my body." Many times, this is very true; they can walk and talk like the rest of us. They are just not able to process there is something wrong with their minds. I try to explain it to them, "You just need more help because you have short term memory problems. That line works like ... almost never. They do not remember that they do not remember. Okay, well, I could tell them how lucky they are not to have to cook or clean again for the rest of their lives! A dream come true for most of us—being waited on forever may get me a moment of reconsideration. Then, they remind me they would rather have their independence. In other words, there is no good answer really, to satisfy Grandma or Gramps. I humbly back out of the room, pull out my prescription pad and start handing out the good stuff. Sometimes, Xanax is the only alternative for the moment.

The Dinner and Scoot Trick

There are other ways of ending up in a nursing home besides the fall and hip fracture route. You can voluntarily move in (which is less common), or you can be basically tricked into the move. It is a bit tough, but at times a necessary technique. It goes like this, "Hey mom, we are just visiting and eating dinner at this new place up the street." Well, once they get in the building, then the family scoots out the back door after dinner. I am the one who is called to see them after, as they are furious. The dinner and scoot trick generally only happens to elderly who are too confused to live alone. Despite the memory loss, they always seem to remember they were tricked. I guess it is true what they say about attaching a strong emotion to an event—you remember it much better. Unfortunately, there really are few ways to convince confused people to even step foot in a home besides a trick. Eventually they will forget what happened, but it can be a bumpy ride.

"The Help-Rejecting Complainer": Victims and Survivors

I am sure everyone in the family is worried over how Grandma will adjust. It's a hard time for all. The staff really will try to get them involved in activities and the life of the home, if the resident allows it. I have also noticed that how well a person adjusts to a nursing home seems to be partially related to whether they were a lifelong optimist or a lifelong pessimist. The pessimist will find that everything you do to try and make them happy becomes a total waste of time. In psychiatry, we call it the "help-rejecting complainer." For those residents, it is better to just listen to all the ways they hate things and then just empathize with their plight. It is okay to say "uncle" when you run up against a constant complainer. What makes it particularly difficult is the unhappy resident may repeat the same negative comment over and over, as if it were the first time. People will even do better if they are not only optimists, but if they have also have been lifelong survivors. I find that in every situation in life, no matter what age, you are either going to be a survivor or a victim of circumstance. So practice when you are young to be an optimist and a survivor. You can see how it will come in handy later if someone "invites you to dinner" at Tropical Oasis. Survivors will always strive to be the survivor, even with dementia.

The "Therapeutic Fiblet"

The adjustment is clearly more difficult if you have memory issues and poor frontal lobe function. Caregivers and staff will be asked hundreds of times, "When am I leaving?" by the resident. I am going to give you a quick trick about how to handle those repeated questions. If you answer that question truthfully, you will agitate the heck out of someone. No one really wants to hear the reality they are loosing all their independence. Well, there is an alternative to telling the truth. It's a technique I learned from a coworker called the "therapeutic fiblet." In other words, you lie. What! You said you couldn't lie? Oh, nurses, staff, and family will learn to do it for their survival. Guilt has no place in this problem. Think about it: if you tell the truth, frontal lobes of the dementia patient really can't process it. They will probably forget what you said that upset them. One could spend hours explaining to a resident why they need to move—and—it's forgotten in ten minutes. I sadly have watched families who stink at lying struggle with this issue. They will explain and re-explain to Grandma how she falls too much, isn't cleaning her house, or is unable to take her medications correctly. Grandma will say, "Yes I can, yes I can, and you can eat off my floors they are so clean." You get nowhere, and you all are annoyed with each other.

Let me give you an example of a therapeutic fiblet to make it clear. What do you say to Grandma when you catch her telling someone that Grandpa will be home soon from work? Now add in the fact that Grandpa has been dead for ten years. Do you say,

"Grandma, we buried Grandpa years ago"? Then you feel horrible as you just made Grandma cry as if she had just heard the news for the first time. We do not really want her to grieve repeatedly. The better alternative is to lie. As far as you know, Grandpa is really out shopping for groceries, wink wink. Lie I tell you, call it a therapeutic fiblit if it makes you feel less guilty. It's a skill that will serve you well. Be creative. So now let's practice with the above example. Think of a lie to tell someone they can't go home. You can make up anything, like there is some kind of water damage to the house and it's not safe to return home. If I were the one being locked up, I would rather it be due to a damaged house than that I can't handle living alone.

There is one other technique besides all out lying for those whose who have trouble lying for various reasons. It is learning how to phrase questions. I learned that one the hard way. Being raised to be polite, I would always ask people as I was leaving, "Do you need anything before I go?" I had kicked myself several times for this, as I ended up getting people more frustrated. Even my kids know I am pretty inadequate at giving them everything they want. For almost every resident I asked if they needed anything, they would respond, "Yes, you can get me home." Now, I was backed into a corner! The best I could come up with in response, "Is there anything else you would like besides going home, as that is not possible?" I really just wanted know if they wanted a drink or something. Now I have to somehow explain why I can't take them home, all for just trying to be nice. Never ever ask an open-ended question. You have to be direct. Now I just say, "Have a nice evening." One more example to solidify my point. What if you need a resident to shower, and they do not want to go with you. Do you say, "We are going to take a shower now," or, "Do you want to shower now?" One option gives them a chance to say no to the shower. Keep it simple and direct.

Assisted Living Facilities

If you are not quite ready to move Mom into a nursing home, we have less scary alternatives. They are called assisted living facilities (ALF). I used to work at the higher end, assisted living facilities in Palm Beach. These places look like hotels, at least they like to give that appearance. They have much cheaper and smaller ALFs as well. The quality of these facilities varies greatly. If Grandma can at least walk and do the minimum in self-care, she can move into her own ALF. They are also much cheaper than a nursing home.

After having worked in them for a time, I can tell you they are great alternatives for a nursing home. Of course, they are appropriate only if Grandma does not require a great deal of physical care. They even have dementia specific ALFs for those who wander.

"I don't want to be around all these 'old people'"

There must be some downside to ALFs of course. These places sound too good to be true. Mom doesn't have to live in a nursing home! Yes, well that is actually the downside—that people move into ALFs that really belong in nursing homes. This leads to a difficult situation within the ALF. The residents who are "with it" notice the residents who appear really confused or physically disabled. This triggers a lot of complaints among the "with it's," as people don't really want to see debilitated people in their homes. "Why are these people here? They belong in a nursing home," I will start hearing. "I don't want to be around all these "old people." You would think this is a small issue, but it's not at all. It's like a mini civil war, except one side doesn't notice there is a war. I have had several odd conversations with elderly residents, who think other people are older than them. I have even heard this argument from eighty-year-olds. Apparently, looking old is really a relative term. One might want to ask Grandma why she has not noticed she is old, but your own frontal lobe stops you. The scene for this where this battle seems to be the most fraught is in the dining room. A person who is "with it" may tell a confused person to stop a certain behavior, for instance, if they are blowing their nose at the table. You will suddenly hear a loud argument as the table fight begins. The confused person takes offense and then words or fists can be exchanged. Some confused residents can yell pretty loud and ruin meals. I have been asked to help the facility make certain elderly residents' behavior is more appropriate in the dining room. I have also been asked to see residents after a physical brawl over such things as seating arrangements. It can be a free for all.

So the issue becomes, how do we help older people not notice they are around old people. Apparently, we have such issues with aging that it has become a task at some places. I had one assisted living facility ban wheelchairs in the lobby and dining room. I know! Hard to believe. Wheelchairs apparently do not make good decor items and remind you of your location. I had one nursing home named Slippery Slope that had a more serious dilemma. There was a group of four wheelchair grannies—Mary, Betty, Joan, and

Nancy—always sitting in the main entrance. The Slippery Slope administrator was hell bent on moving them out of there. Why, you ask? Mary, Betty, Joan, and Nancy would sit and gossip for hours. Apparently they had good enough hearing to find out some juicy gossip from the staff that would pass by them. I mean come on; eavesdropping was way more fun than bingo. But apparently, they were considered an eye sore to the public touring the building. Eventually, the Slippery Slope "four" lost the battle and were moved to a less obvious location. I miss those little ladies. I was always tempted to tell them a false rumor and see how far it would spread.

At least Mary, Betty, Joan, and Nancy were fun. I could better understand why another home banned certain residents from the lobby of my home called Secret Hideaway. I will never forget asking one family member named Patricia why she did not pick Secret Hideaway to send her mother, Margaret. This is what she said. "I was walking in the front entrance, and a guy asked me for a blow job." I can appreciate her being hesitant now that she explained. I was never able to figure out which resident said that line to Patricia. Trust me, I was dying to know. Unfortunately, doing a police-style line up with the residents was not allowed. You just think little old Bill is out there getting some fresh air, and the next thing you know, he is hitting on visitors. Secret Hideaway then built a sitting area spaced away from the front entrance for the residents. Ban Bill and his buddies from the lobby? Heck no, they just hide them better. Now the guys had to sit far to the left of the front lobby. I suppose they still could cat call a good-looking visitor still from that distance.

Making a Run for It

Speaking of main entrances, there is another issue related to them: residents trying to elope from the building. You just never know when you will get that call that they found Charles down at the local store trying to buy cigarettes. It is also impossible to predict who is going to try to make a run for it. I mean, the nursing homes try to predict. We have these little forms with checkboxes to show we at least attempt to find the potential elopers. It helps us sleep better at night. The elopers are usually those with dementia of course. But we never expected this from Charles! Paul and Jack, perhaps. If a resident dings positive on our eloper scale, then they are tagged a "wander risk." The nurse then applies a leg brace to the resident. I suppose it looks something similar to house arrest.

I have several confused residents who ask why they have to wear the ugly thing on their ankle. Of course the quick and dirty answer is, "In case you try to escape from here, a loud alarm will sound or the door will lock. Apparently, they do not trust you to stay in here without an ankle brace." Since this answer never seems to go over well, sometimes we have to throw out a fiblet. The best one I have seen is a nurse telling a resident that the bracelet is actually a heart monitor. I give her kudos for that one. For those who are still persistent enough to leave, they figure out how to cut the bracelet off. I had one guy named John who was a carpenter prior to developing dementia. He was really good at getting the alarm off. He was also trying to take apart everything else in his room. John was tough!

If the leg alarms do not stop you, then it's the locked unit for you. Yes, you are already closed in a nursing home and then locked in again behind doors. The main entrance doors are not always completely secured. People find ways out of the main entrance when someone has their back turned. My home even had pictures like mug shots of all the potential elopers posted over the nursing stations. Sometimes the residents looked so much like visitors, we could be fooled. Moving to the locked unit can be traumatic of course. There is that horrible stage of dementia where you are "with it" enough to elope, but not confused enough to realize you were just locked in a dementia unit. You are now surrounded by really, really confused people, including many who can't even hold a logical conversation. The only way out is by knowing the code on the door or slipping out behind someone exiting. I do not think I have to explain how being on the unit upsets the eloper. It can make the families even more upset. We all know it's not the ideal location for the person, but we have to keep them safe until there is a better option.

This is why I have been asked to evaluate people who were threatening to walk out. The home wanted my opinion whether I felt the person was an elopement risk. It is to avoid these horrible situations. If the resident would continue to threaten to leave with me, I would do what any highly trained psychiatrist would do. I would beg. "Please don't try to leave. I know what they will do to you. You will end up on the locked unit!" I warned. Yes, I can safely say my warnings never worked. If you are threatening to leave, and you have poor frontal lobe function, then you need a more secure unit. Families would be irate with us at times because we suggest a locked unit. "My Mom is not demented like those other people."

It honestly is a horrible situation. This is why I tried begging the person not to leave. I knew begging would not help me escape the situation, but it made me feel better for a minute. The nursing homes do not want the liability of a lost resident, so it can become a battle between the home and the family. This is another example of making the best possible decision out of several bad options.

I was always surprised when those families did not remove their "eloper" from the home if they hated the unit so much. Sometimes families do not have that option to move their loved one. The decisions sometimes come down to how much money they have to spend. If you have the money, you can pay privately for a locked ALF or private duty nurse at home 24/7. As you may know, Medicaid pays the cost of nursing homes, so they are affordable. This is after you spend down most of your savings. Medicaid, on the other hand, may only pay a portion of the cost of an ALF. Your social security and your savings will cover the rest of the bill. The more money you have to spend, the better the options. Did I tell you all that I put as much as I can in my IRA? I want a locked unit in Trump Tower if I have to go to one. Sunset Manor, one of the smarter locked ALFs in town, separated out the residents based on levels of severity of their dementia. This prevented the more "with it" residents from being blended with the extremely confused residents. People really adjusted much better with this small change. We all need to get more creative as this home has done.

I know many families feel forced into moving a family member to a locked unit, and I totally understand. They are fighting for the sanity of their loved ones. But the public does not always get to see the bad consequences of elopement from the medical staff's point of view. I had an older man (sad story alert) elope from the home and drowned in one of the many canals winding around Florida buildings. One woman eloped, and even helicopters couldn't locate her. They eventually found her in a tree outside the nursing home. The payout to the family was pretty good I hear, because they lost her. Some homes will ask families to move the potential elopers out due to the potential liability. I suppose when you know every possible bad outcome, you think locked units are the not the worst alternative. Death and injury are clearly much worse. We had a woman, Dorothy, who kept trying to elope down a stairway in her wheelchair. I can't even imagine what that injury looked like. A locked unit seems less awful if you think in those terms. At least the family can know their loved one is safe until we can all rethink possible solutions.

Wandering Inside the Home

Just when wandering couldn't sound worse, we have residents who wander *inside* the building. They are not trying to leave; they just become lost. Yes, even they are a problem as innocent as this sounds. I worked at a home called Jolly Rancher with a guy named Charlie. His room to room wandering got Jolly Rancher in big trouble with the state. How? Charlie wandered into a female resident's room uninvited. Charlie had to pee and her bathroom was the closest he could find. Of course, the woman thought he was coming in for something even more indecent. Apparently, Charlie inadvertently violated not only this woman's rights by invading her privacy. He also mentally traumatized her per the State of Florida. The home was penalized with a "tag," an official black mark on their record. Well, after this, the home no longer was willing to accept wandering residents for fear of liability. This is one of the reasons why I am asked to see the "victims" of wanderers for any signs of possible abuse. I was not asked to see this woman to know how traumatized she was by Charlie. The state made the decision before I was asked to give my input. Charlie's wife was asked to move him from the building after the incident. It was a sad resolution for us all. I now find it harder and harder to find a locked unit that is not fearful of backlash. Many are closing in my area.

"I'll Beat the Crap Out of Her"

So, even the confused residents are not allowed to wander? I was getting really confused about what confused residents could do. Imagine how confused they must feel. Wanderers will always wander in the homes; it is just a reality family and staff have to face. Wanderers will get into other's belongings, steal other resident's clothes, get in their beds. They may even relieve themselves in other's air conditioning units. Their frontal lobes are simply not processing information correctly. I had a patient named Charlotte once who really put this issue in an interesting perspective. She had a chronic mental illness as well as a dementia developing—a double whammy. She, like many mentally ill, would hoard her belongings in her room. It looked like a giant garage sale all the time. It was so tempting for others to want to browse the junk pile. Well, she had this one woman down the hall—Gail—that she hated. There was a battle between them after Gail started hunting for treasure. Gail was always wandering into Charlotte's room until finally, punches were thrown. This is always the time when the psychiatrist gets called in to assess the "danger." Charlotte let me know very bluntly that she would beat the "crap" out of Gail if she returned. Of course, I told her what any logical person would say, "If you hit her, you will be in trouble." I know, profound advice. I had to pay off over 100K in student loans to get that profound. Well, Charlotte was smart enough to let me know that she could get away with bruising up Gail. "Who are they going to believe? She is too confused to report me." Charlotte was good, still "with it" enough to plan a beat down and get away with it. Well, since once again there were no drugs that could solve this problem, we had to have Plan B again. I asked for the large stop signs made for this purpose. They are velcroed across a resident's doorway. Not sure why we don't use them more. A good home will invest in them. So, we did just that. The bright red stop sign scared Gail off. Gail was confused enough at that point to fall for it. Thank goodness as Charlotte looked like a real scrapper.

Sex?

Well, I know you have all been waiting for me to discuss sex in the nursing home. Getting older does not take away your urges for sure. What do you do if two confused people want to date, or even consummate the relationship? We have to first see if they are competent to consent. Of course, many are not, and these are the ones I get called to see. If they are NOT competent, then the families gets to be the lucky ones to decide if Mom can hold hands, kiss, and all that other stuff people do. Sometimes, two elderly people will just gravitate to each other and keep each other company. The families say it is fine, everyone is happy. Of course, this clearly is not how it always ends up. I get sucked into bad situations and dread these consults. What if one of the two family members does not want the affair to continue. For example, I had one married man named Peter who was a new resident in my home. His wife would visit daily, and when she would go home for the night, the fun would begin. Peter fell in love with another confused female resident, Mary. They became inseparable. It was not even anything beyond hand holding. The wife would return the next day to find Peter with Mary. All hell broke loose, and I was instructed by the wife to do all we could to keep them apart. He was a married man for goodness sake! In her mind he was cheating. Of course, Peter didn't understand at all and would become aggressive when we tried to separate him from

Mary. He must have thought of Mary as his real wife now. Obviously, it was an impossible task. We had to try to convince the wife it was not really cheating if Peter was confused. Sadly, it all fell on deaf ears. I told them there was no way I could medicate Peter to stay away from Mary. The only way to solve the issue was for one to relocate. As it happened, Peter died soon after, and I was saved a horrible battle. I think if Peter's wife understood dementia better, she would not have objected. Peter had found some quality of life in a horrible situation. He was so calm and happy when he held his girlfriend's hand. I know this is not how his wife imagined their relationship ending. I'm sure it was traumatic for her, but it really wasn't personal. Peter really was not cheating. He would have to remember he was married in the first place. There are numerous other scenarios, but I wanted to give you an idea so you all can mentally prepare yourself for Mom stepping out again.

Sexual Aggression

Obviously, not all relationships are consensual. Some male residents are sexually assaultive. It is *very scary* for all involved when this happens. I really only have a few options to resolve the situation. One is moving a resident to an all male unit. I wish we had one in my county. To be honest, I have only seen one all male home. It was a home for demented Catholic priests in New Hampshire. I hate to say it, but even the male priests were also sexually aggressive to each other. I don't want to even think what that was all about. So an all male unit is unlikely to happen. Okay, so the other option is basically chemical castration. There is a medical way to lower your testosterone levels so you are safe to be around women. It sounds almost barbaric, but what do we do with sexually aggressive men? I hate this part of the job. I hate it so much, I am ending this paragraph NOW.

Paranoia: A Trigger for Fear and Violence

There is one symptom that up to one-half off all people with dementia develop: paranoia. This symptom keeps me very busy. Let me first define what a paranoid delusion is. Paranoid delusions are a fixed false belief, not based in reality. For example, your eighty-year-old husband accusing you of prostituting yourself for money would be considered a delusion. This, of course, is assuming you are not really a prostitute. Other delusions are conspiracy theories involving nurses. For example, they will tell me the nurses are passing medications to run experiments on residents. Even today I asked a resident why he was so afraid of the nurse. "She is in on the sham here. Whisper until she leaves the room." He did not even believe she was his nurse at all. Many confuse paranoid delusions with a person who is just plain confused. It is important to understand the difference, as the treatment is different. I gave an example of a woman who was having a relationship with her deceased husband. It could qualify as a delusions as it is a false, fixed belief not based in reality. It is, however, more like simple confusion, as she is not able to recall that her husband died. It was a happy confused thought for her. I would not treat it with medications or argue with her. The true paranoid delusions, on the other hand, need to be treated with medications. Why? Because paranoia triggers both fear and violence. It is the main cause of violence in my opinion. Those living in paranoia generally do not have a good quality of life. This is why I tend to treat the symptom with medication.

Since we want to prevent violence, you all need to be taught how to catch paranoia. I will give you a few tips. It actually is not always easy to notice. Paranoid people do not trust you, so why should they tell you the conspiracy in their head. You might be one of the people trying to harm them. For me, I have to diagnose paranoia rather quickly. If I don't, things could escalate into violence. First, there is the straightforward approach. Every now and then, I get lucky by using my innocent Indiana charm and just ask them straight up, "Are you afraid anyone is trying to hurt you? You tell me who that person is, and I will take care of them immediately." You have to look as harmless as possible, and you may even want to sit lower than them. If the direct approach fails, you can try the casual conversation. Make the patient think you are one of them. For instance, "I see a lot of things happen in this place. Do any of these nurses give you problems?" This statement has opened up a few paranoid people to tell me the nurses were poisoning them. This is why they were trying to beat them up during medication pass. The last but not least technique I have is to ask the janitors, activity staff, or aides if they have heard anything odd that the person may have said in passing. In one home, the Cuban maintenance guy I worked with gave me all the dirt on the Latino residents. He let me know one Latin male thought the communists were going to invade the home soon. I would have never known that without the custodian. I have my secret eyes and ears around the building, and so should you!

I do have one quality that tends to naturally trigger paranoia I am looking to find. I smile all the time. People even refer to me as "that doctor who is always smiling." My rap name is Dr. Smile-a-lot. My Asian name is "woman with big choppers." I think you get my point. What do you want? My mother always said, "Let your smile be your umbrella." Apparently, I took it a little too far. I have had more than one person say, "Are you laughing at me?" I guess my personal quality has come in handy as a psychiatrist. Smile at a paranoid person long enough, and they are going to talk. I obviously do not recommend this as a real technique. I am really not trying it intentionally and have had to curb my grin over the years.

Psychosis

Next to paranoia, there is one more symptom that we group with the general term, "psychosis." You can always be classified as psychotic if you are having either visual or auditory hallucinations. You see things no one else sees, or you hear things when no one is around. I see this issue the most with those suffering from Parkinson's disease/Parkinson's dementia. They have the most vivid visual hallucinations possible. They will describe to me very clear pictures of the hallucinations. One man, for instance, told me he saw people ballroom dancing outside his window. He actually loved it, so I was not concerned too much. They also can have very vivid dreams or vivid nightmares. Many are very distressed by the nightmares. One thing that few people may know, the medications we use to treat Parkinson's disease can cause you to hallucinate. Medications such as Sinemet, Mirapex, and Requip—you would think they were like legal LSD. Every time I see a person with Parkinson's, I ask if they have nightmares or hallucinations. Sometimes, they are too afraid to mention it, as it is embarrassing. Once I tell them it is part of the illness, they feel relieved and hopeful I can help them. Besides Parkinson's disease, one other illness, Lewy Body dementia, is known for causing visual hallucinations. Lewy Body dementia has many other similarities to Parkinson's disease, but I would refer you to read other sources if you are interested in knowing more about this illness.

Violence in the Home

Again, psychosis is so important for me *not* to miss, as it's a real trigger for violence. I want to do all I can to prevent injuries, so

I feel it as even more urgent to find its cause. I have been asked multiple times to see a resident who was recently violent. I get there as quickly as possible, only to find the aggressor being calm and charming. The nurses look at me annoyed. They remind me I only visit when everyone is on their best behavior. People seem to change minute to minute. Of course, the calm silence after the storm also fools families who receive the same call that their parent was aggressive. Since they do not always see it with their own eyes, they sometimes do not believe the nurses' reports. I swear, the families only seem to visit when Mom is being nice as well. It is so frustrating. Again, I wish I could walk away and pretend everything is good. I can avoid having to explain to the family how I had to medicate Grandma for hitting, when they think I must have the wrong person. The family will not believe it, and the nurses let me know I have to do something before someone is injured. I am caught in the middle.

How do you solve this problem? Well, I personally want to see the aggression before I give someone medication. I owe it to the patient and the family. To personally witness the aggression, you have to get creative. I encourage families to do the same if you are having trouble believing the nurses. If you really really want to know Grandma, visit her at night.

Sundowning

Like Halloween, all bad things seem to come out after the sun sets. Unlike Halloween, we do not call it the bewitching hour, we call it "sundowning." That little cute nugget is all sweet until about 5 p.m. The family goes home. "I'll see you tomorrow Mom." Everyone is happy and smiling. The clock hits 6 p.m. and the same nugget is throwing chairs in the dining room. The nurse calls to notify the family they need to give her medications. The family thinks they are calling the wrong family, as there is no way it is their Mom. Eventually, the family is able to see the aggression, and the medical staff and the families can work together to find solutions. Of course every family is different; some readily accept the need to control the aggression. They do not want anyone injured. Some families place the blame of the aggression on the staff. They feel the staff is provoking the aggression, or that the staff is just not trained well enough to prevent aggression. I am sure this *is* the case at times. So what to do to figure out who is at fault? I can just tell you what I do to unravel the puzzle. I listen to all sides of the story including my own exam. Then I look to see if Mom is consistently aggressive with everyone. Is she an equal opportunity hitter? Then Mom is looking guiltier. I also look for any physical injuries to staff or peers from Mom. I understand residents verbally losing their tempers with inexperienced staff, but it if is escalating to the point of physical violence, then the resident may have serious impulse control problems. Once again, the frontal lobe is not kicking in. Sometimes, it is impossible to know the actual situation with conflicting stories. If I am not sure, then I just re-evaluate the situation over time to be sure. I do not want to medicate someone who does not require it.

I have one other trick up my sleeve to see aggression in potentially violent residents. I don't like to pull it out unless I have to do so. There are times I have to decide whether to send a person to the hospital due to aggression. Most of the time, I show up after the event is over, and the resident is calm. I have panicked nurses telling me to send them out. I want to be fair and see the anger with my own eyes. I listen to nurses' reports. I see if any damage is done, bruises and so forth, I speak to the resident who generally say, "They are all liars." They will not even recall the incident most of the time. I can't leave a potentially violent guy to strike again after I leave. I prefer he lose his cool at me instead of a little old lady after I go home. So I do what I have to do to get the information I need. So, I try to piss the person off myself. It is not hard for me to do—I have been a little sister all my life. I have skills. You basically start a circular argument. You want to see if they can hold their temper. It gives me a good idea of their frustration tolerance. Desperate times lead to desperate measures. Obviously, no one else should try this move. I only do it to test people. It is just one more bit of evidence I have to help me make a good decision. I would rather have them punch me than anyone else. The nurses that know me well get what I am doing; others may find me a bit unusual. All I can say is, "I get the job done."

Depression and Delirium

I do have to mention a few other major issues that can arise before I close this chapter. Depression and delirium. Let's start with delirium. Delirium is basically confusion triggered by medical issues. Specifically, delirium is a waxing and waning of consciousness. You are clear and logical one minute, and the next you are trying to kill bugs crawling up the wall. Hallucinations, mainly visual, can be prominent.

Paranoia is also a common finding. You can also have severe disorientation. They also sometimes refer to delirium as ICU psychosis. The biggest causes: infection and anesthesia/surgery. I am not sure if it is the anesthesia or pain medications that cause the confusion, or the shifts in blood pressure from a surgery. No one totally knows why elderly come out of surgery extremely confused and fighting. I am called to medicate the person so they do not injure themselves or others. I can tell you that you need to ask the surgeon how high are the risks of delirium before your loved one has surgery. One thing they do not emphasize to you during the consents is the risk that your elderly family member may have a decline in their cognitive ability after the surgery. In other words, someone with just mild to no memory issues prior to the surgery can develop symptoms of dementia after the surgery. Delirium can be a predictor of this future decline. You sometimes have to wait up to six months to know if the confusion from the delirium will fully clear. The risk seems to be the highest in heart surgeries, probably because you need that blood to be reaching the brain. Hip and knee surgeries can be the culprit as well. I just need people to be aware of the surgery risks, especially after the age of eighty. As many of the nurses will tell me, "They saved his heart, but they sure messed up his brain."

Last but not least, I am called to treat anxiety and depression—the meat and potatoes of psychiatry. Interestingly, the most common response from the residents when I am asked to see them for depression is, "Wouldn't you be depressed if you were here?" Ah yes, I would be down. I, however, am not referring to this type of depression. I am looking for a real depression. Most people are naturally upset they are in a nursing home. If you just want to vent about the food or the aides, I will send the nurse back in to listen. That is their job. No, I am joking—I love to tease nurses. It is not that this initial adjustment depression is not important, I just have to be able to spot the depressions that will cause some damage. Depression is a big cause of treatment failures. Depressed people refuse more physical therapy, do not eat well, and generally adjust poorly. Depression can even make residents appear as if they have dementia.

I need to describe to you what you will have to look for to diagnose this potentially devastating illness. Depression is defined as depressed and/or irritable mood for more days than not. It usually has to be at least for a few weeks before we can make the diagnosis. I emphasize irritable, as sometimes, the irritability is more prominent than the depressed mood. I have had people tell me they do not actually feel depressed, they just want to snap at everyone. Once you find the mood changes, you can look at other possible symptoms like loss of interest, loss of the ability to experience pleasure, increased negativity, poor self image, increased guilt (especially of being a burden to others), hopelessness, and suicidal ideation. The suicidal thoughts can be on a continuum of just feeling ready to die, to doing things to increase your risk of death (refusing to eat or take medications), to actually planning on harming yourself. You can also see loss of appetite and decreased or increased ability to sleep. These are called vegetative symptoms of depression. These are not always as reliable a predictor of depression, as many medical illnesses cause appetite and sleep issues as well.

What many people do not realize is that a significant depression is one of the first signs of dementia. I have seen it over and over again. You will have that person who has never really been a depressed person in the past. They start having depression for the first time in their seventies and eighties. I am not sure why dementia triggers a depression beyond the changing brain chemistry and brain cell loss. It is obviously not what I want to tell a depressed person, that they have early dementia. I usually try to see if I can treat the depression and see how much memory improves. There is actually what we call "pseudo dementia" meaning that someone looks so depressed that they struggle with memory and concentration problems. It is not a real dementia. But in my experience, most often the case is that they have early dementia.

Apathy

There is one other symptom that can be confused with depression. It is actually another one of those darned frontal lobe issues. Your frontal lobe is important to help with drive and motivation. I am repeatedly asked to see residents with no motivation. They will sit all day and show no desire to get up, leave the room, go to therapy, and even do self-care. It is actually called the syndrome of apathy. Apathy is confused all the time with depression, but it is not the same. An apathetic person will not describe any symptoms of depression. They are perfectly happy doing nothing. It is actually their spouse who is the one complaining the most. It is hard, as most people just see it as laziness, but it is actually not the same at all. Some wives get so mad with their husband's immobility that they threaten to divorce them. It is a total damper on your social life. We all have moments of apathy but generally not daily. There are certain medications that help it the most, usually the ones that raise norepinephrine or brain dopamine. These chemicals are responsible for that sense of drive and motivation. We even try Ritalin, which you all know we use for children with attention issues. Sometimes it even works. The goal is to improve quality of life.

Conclusion

I think I have given you a pretty good look into all the issues that come up for me. I will give more examples later when I describe a typical day. I did decide to devote the next chapter to the medications. I see how badly families struggle to understand what medications do—the pros and cons. They are actually hard to figure out, and you may get several different opinions. It will hopefully guide you through a future conversation with your doctor about the issue. I will be honest about the limitations of medications. I wish drugs fixed all the issues. I do think they take the edge off of many problems. Dementia is a brain disease, and there is no pill to fix your brain. It does not regenerate like a liver or skin cell. As I will continue to repeat, with dementia you are trying to improve quality of life. If a medication can improve quality without having uncomfortable side effects, then you have accomplished a great deal. Since dementia is a brain disease that can show changes in either mood or behavior, you can also ask a neurologist for help as well. Dementia is, after all, a "neuropsychological" illness. Many times, neurologists handle the behavioral symptoms. You can find either a good neurologist or a geriatric psychiatrist to help. You will just happen to see more psychiatrists hanging out in nursing homes, so apparently you are stuck with us.

━━━━ CHAPTER 5 ━━━━

Pills, Pills, Pills

- ➤ Neurotransmitters.
- ➤ Antidepressants.
- ➤ Serotonin, norepinephrine, and dopamine.
- ➤ Tranquilizers.
- ➤ Addiction and interdose rebound.
- ➤ Falls.
- ➤ Paradoxical reactions.
- ➤ Aggressive behavior and medications.
- ➤ Antipsychotics.

Are you ready to conquer the world of medications? How do all these medications even work anyhow? How can a pill even change mood and behavior? You need to first understand how the brain cells work.

Neurotransmitters

The brain cells are full of chemicals called neurotransmitters. Neurotransmitters are how the cells communicate with each other. Think of it like squeezing a tube of toothpaste. Imagine your fingers as the medication, the brain cells are the tube of paste, the neurotransmitters are the toothpaste, and the teeth are the other brain cells getting the message. We want to get out every last drop of toothpaste out of the cell and this is the job of the antidepressants. The medications cause the cells to shower the neurotransmitters all over each other. This sounds a bit too much like a weird sex scene! Sorry! Serotonin, norepinephrine, and dopamine are the toothpaste of the cells. They are the main neurotransmitters. Not to simplify the issue, but these chemicals can control our moods and behaviors.

These neurotransmitters are also the basis for several of our theories on depression and anxiety. Depressed people seem to be deficient in these neurotransmitters. This is at least one theory to explain why increasing our brain serotonin can actually help lower anxiety and depression. When I first started prescribing medications, I actually was pretty nervous. I had a hard time believing that this theory would work. Then I saw really sad people get back into their groove. Of course, nothing is a panacea, but it was at least something. When you see enough mental suffering, I was ready to use pills.

When to Prescribe a New Pill

I take every decision to start a medication very seriously, as if each person were my own family. There sometimes is an unspoken pressure on doctors to always prescribe "something." Some people seem to want to leave the doctor's office with a script in their hands. It's what we do as doctors—we write scripts and order tests. This is obviously not true in every situation, but we have to recognize when this force is in play. It reminds me when my four-year-old daughter sees me take a Motrin for a headache. The next thing you know, she needs a Motrin for her headache. Before that, she had no idea what a headache was, but it looks like fun to take a pill. Now I tell my daughter she does not have enough stress to have a headache or a pill, and then I go take my pill in secret. Bottom line, I just refuse to prescribe unneeded medications to anyone. I am the first to cry "uncle" when I know a pill is useless. For example, I have had several consults for residents spitting on floors. It is just a bad habit unrelated to chewing tobacco. Spitting is also an obvious safety hazard, as well as a really gross habit. There is no medication that will stop spitting. I accept defeat in this situation and humbly walk away—over the spit puddle hopefully. With all this said, I still see a great deal of conflict about the use of medication in nursing homes between doctors, nurses, families, and sometimes even the patients. There is a constant discussion on what we give, to whom we give it, and why it is needed at all. I am hoping to decrease the stress of these arguments with a solid explanation of the medications.

K-Pins, Zannies, and Xanbars!

There are four main classes of medications we can use for the various problems we encounter: antidepressants, tranquilizers, antipsychotics, and seizure medications. I am actually asked by residents and nurses the most to prescribe the tranquilizers, so I will start with them. I am forever trying to talk people out of these medications. I lately have even started to cringe when I hear the names of these drugs—Ativan, Xanax, Valium, and Klonopin. Ugh! My dread has only grown worse as I have started working in drug treatment centers, and I am learning all the street names for these pills. Klonopin is called K-Pins and Xanax are Zanniesor Xanbars. Sometimes ignorance is bliss, like I really did not have to find out people can snort them too. They are addictive obviously and have a street value. Many innocent grandmothers have had their prescription medications stolen, so hide them well. In my training, we were told to refer to these meds as "alcohol in a pill." My teachers were correct—they act in the brain the same way as alcohol. Personally, I would rather drink my alcohol. With the many types of flavored vodka, why would anyone choose a pill? Of course, we do not have alcohol in the nursing home, so the choice is easy. The only facility I have seen with a bar was an assisted living facility. Everyone was calm and relaxed at night, even though the bartender was always watering down the drinks. So the Xanax pill or the rum punch? Still a hotly debated issue.

Tranquilizers are also called sedative-hypnotics or benzodiazepines, just so you are all well rounded with the terms we use. The problems with these medications are several. These medications can lead to what is called tolerance. This means, it takes more and more medication to have the same calming effect if you take them on a regular basis. The body has this amazing trick of always trying to bring you back to your original state. The liver learns how to process the medications faster so they are gone quicker. You lose the original calming effect and are then wanting more.

Most people can relate to alcohol, so I will use it as an example. Say you have a few beers a day and you want to go get a drink with a friend who drinks once a month. You can drink much more and stay longer at the bar. Your friend is ready to sleep under the bar with the same amount. As a result, you do not ask that friend to drink with you again. All kidding aside, as doctors, we know tolerance easily develops. We dread that request to keep increasing a person's Xanax dose because the current dose is not working. We fear it may lead to the eventual abuse of Xanax.

The other issues with tranquilizers are that they cause physical and psychological dependence. I have detoxed hundreds of people off these medications and trust me, it's a difficult experience. You are not only mentally craving the medication, but you may also be experiencing physical symptoms as your body tries to readjust to being without the medication. Withdrawal occurs as your body is trying to return to how it was working before you ever took the Xanax. This is a simple explanation of withdrawal. Let me give you an example. When I was in medical school, we were called to see a man who was trying to basically beat the crap out of the nurses. He was three days out of a surgery. We had to restrain him quickly before we were punched. What had happened to him was that his doctor did not restart his tranquilizer after his surgery was over. He was accidentally forced into a tranquilizer withdrawal at its worst. Rapid heart rate, high blood pressures, tremors, sweats, and severe anxiety were all the symptoms. Of course, not every person is going to need to be strapped to a bed in a withdrawal! This case is an extreme example. Your particular withdrawal symptoms depend on how addicted you are to the medication.

What? I've Got Interdose Rebound Withdrawal!

There is a less known issue with tranquilizers called "interdose rebound" withdrawal. It is basically withdrawal anxiety in between your doses of Xanax. Hold on tight—this is complicated. A patient comes in to see a doctor because they feel anxious. The doctor starts them on Xanax for their anxiety. The person may have to take it up to two to three times a day, as it really only lasts about four hours in their blood. The medications are then keeping the patient happy, feeling calmer, and he or she thinks the problem is solved. Oh no! It is just beginning! Follow me here. Xanax is a short-acting tranquilizer. The shorter a drug lasts in your system, the more quickly you will start to notice the withdrawal symptoms from it. Its main withdrawal symptom is anxiety. You can feel the anxiety increase as the body is quickly getting the Xanax out of your system. So in between Xanax doses, you are having these mini withdrawals. You take the medication at 8 a.m. and by noon you are experiencing the beginnings of a withdrawal. So not only do you have the anxiety you walked in the doctor's office with, but now you are experiencing periods of Xanax withdrawal throughout the day. You are starting to chase a withdrawal of Xanax. I always knew who was having issues with Xanax in my nursing homes, as they would be following the nurses around as the Xanax withdrawal was kicking in. "Is my Xanax due yet? Of course they call it their "little pill." The end result is you feel like a walking yoyo. If they destroyed all Xanax in the world, I would perhaps be the happiest shrink around. If I have to use a tranquilizer, I usually choose the longer acting ones. Examples of longer acting tranquilizers are Ativan and Klonopin.

The Ativanatini, The Valium Chaser, The Klonopin Margarita

As with all things are in life, it is not always so black and white. Tranquilizers do have a select place in the medical field. Yes, the Ativanatini, the Valium Chaser, and the Klonopin margarita can be useful. We just have to be very careful and look at the following: (1) Why exactly are we starting them? (2) What else can we do to help someone's anxiety besides pills; (3) Monitor side effects; and (4) always reevaluate if we can stop them later on. Okay. One more, (5) Do not give high doses, as they probably will not help in the long run. Oh yes, and if a person does think high doses work, they are possibly at risk for abuse of the medication.

Since I am not able to go over every situation when I feel comfortable with using them, maybe I can give a fast summary. There are always going to be some people in nursing homes who feel they can't live without their tranquilizers. The pills may not even be helping at all, but it is the psychological need for them. It gives them some sense of quality, and the fear of stopping them is not worth it. I leave them alone unless they are falling all over with sedation. I like the tranquilizers for diseases that cause shortness of breath and panic-like sensations. Diseases like emphysema (COPD) cause "air hunger" and panic. I also use them if you are adjusting to a loss or a change and need them for the short term. For residents who are fearful or aggressive, these meds can also help. I prefer to use them as needed (PRN) versus given routinely. Less than daily use is the safest. If someone is trying to rip a door off a wall, most definitely give them a shot of the medication. Shot meaning with a needle of course. Just know that overall, tranquilizers are a temporary fix to an issue. Once they wear off, you are back to where you started. I prefer medications that may take some time to work, but are always giving my nuggets a continuous payoff. I have always been better at delayed gratification than the quick fix. Xanax is the quick fix, not my ideal.

A few other side effects to be watchful for as you take tranquilizers. I guess the worst would be abuse of the medication. Abuse is not the same as physical and mental dependence. The following is how I explain abuse of these medications for those fearful of getting "hooked": "unless you are stealing them from others, doctor shopping to get more drugs, just generally not following the instructions on the bottle, then you are probably not abusing them." It would actually be hard to abuse the medication in a nursing home. Fortunately, we have locked medication carts in homes. So this is why you have to pack Mom's lock pick or some type of hairpin in her luggage. Maybe a few quick lessons on picking a lock as well. If she is going to get the "good stuff," it's locked away and she can't abuse it. I have yet to see a successful drug heist, and I am very disappointed with my nuggets. The nurses still steal way more tranquilizers than anyone. Come to think of it, I did have a nurse stash her goods in an elderly person's room. She was trying not to get caught. The nugget later confessed she was hiding them for her nurse. I suppose that does not qualify for a nugget drug heist though. It was close.

Ride the Xanax Train at Your Own Risk

I actually prescribe very few tranquilizers. Many residents come in the homes already on them. Each visit, I get a list of new clients we received from the hospital who are on tranquilizers. I have to ask them, "Do you still need that Ativan? Can we get rid of it for you?" What residents do not always realize is the amount of scrutiny these medications are under in nursing homes. The State of Florida and even Medicare want all these medications evaluated and reduced. We have constant meetings to discuss which resident's medications can be lowered and taken off the orders. The insurance companies even send me letters about the medications they feel need to be stopped. Psychiatric medications are the most scrutinized medications in the home. Medicare even rates the quality of a home based on how many residents are on these medications. Your nursing home star ratings will drop if residents have too many drugs. I wish the government scrutinized other issues as much as they do Grandma's sleeping pill. I was a little bitter about it at first. Not because I do not feel they should be monitored, but because it seems this group of medications are scrutinized more than any other class of drugs. Let's try to stop some blood pressure pills people, maybe even a diabetes medication.

Falls

In addition to the new admits on drugs, the pharmacy sends me a list of sleeping pills and tranquilizers I have to try to stop. "Can I stop your sleeping pill?' I have annoyed many a little elderly person with that question. "Just doing my job here, it's cool," I'll keep it moving," as I have had my head chewed off for asking. I am also asked to see residents who are falling and are taking either sleeping pills or tranquilizers. These meds are clearly linked to fall risk. Many do not want to hear about the falling side effect. If you do not believe me, show me a college freshman that has not fallen after their first party at school. If you can fall from booze, you can fall from pills. I can proudly say, I did not fall until several months into my freshman year in college. I always prided myself in my coordination skills, even when drinking. My fall, of course, was only because I was in freezing Ithaca, NY. There is a lot of black ice there.

I always love to hear the excuses of why residents feel they really fell down. It is never because of the sleeping pills. "My Ambien didn't make me fall. I tripped on the bed." "I fell way after taking that pill." My favorite was a woman who fell and broke a hip after a taking a Xanax and an Ambien together at home. She told me she never actually fell, she was just cleaning the floor and her leg broke spontaneously. I get it lady, you want to stay on your medications. I know you do, but the nursing homes' big fear is you will fall on these medications and then sue them for not preventing the fall. So, if you want them, you have to tell me you understand they will cause falls. We should have them sign a release of liability like you do on those crazy amusement park rides. Ride the Xanax train at your own risk. Nursing homes do not want this liability. Of course, if someone understands the risks and tells me they need the sleep aide to function the next day, I will leave the pill. If you fall again, I feel better you had a heads up first, and I hope that you bounce when you fall and not break anything. When I am old, I may want a sleeping pill too. A restful sleep is at times a nice escape. I try not to go crazy stopping all these sleep aides.

The decision to use Ativan in patients who are extremely agitated and confused is more difficult. You have to weigh multiple variables. Is the resident suffering mentally? Are they going to be a fall risk after taking the medication? There is also the risk that the Ativan can make them even more agitated. This is actually a real phenomenon called a "paradoxical reaction." Sorry! I have to use another drinking analogy—they just are so clear. Despite my many analogies, I do not drink that much. Okay, so you have some friends that get calm and cool after a beer, and then you have those other friends who get loud and obnoxious. Have you ever tried to hide from your drunken friends as they do stupid things? Well, the same is true in the elderly. Ativan can make them angrier and more agitated. When a resident is getting more agitated on Ativan, there are always debates between staff if it is a paradoxical reaction. Should we stop the Ativan as it is making someone worse? The best way to know if it is a paradoxical reaction is to be clear how severe the agitation was before the medication was ever given. What is the exact target symptom you are trying to treat with medication? This could be crying, fearfulness, or hitting. If they are still agitated after the Ativan, it may just mean they did not respond to that particular medication or the dose was too low. If they have increased agitation after the med, maybe they have the paradoxical reaction.

The same idea goes with confusion. Ativan may make you MORE confused. You HAVE to get a baseline level of confusion to know if it is increasing someone's confusion. A big issue I run into is families or nurses claiming the medications made someone confused. Then I look through the chart and it clearly states the person was confused already in the hospital before taking the medications. We have to all agree how confused they were before we start Ativan. In this way, then you know if it was the Ativan that made them confused or the confusion was already present from a medical issue or dementia. This again is why we need to ask all ten questions on the dementia screening. You can never assume someone is alert and oriented unless you ask them specific questions. They will fool you, no matter how well you think you know them.

The Target Symptom

I have to keep emphasizing finding a target symptom. You are better able to tell what is going on if you are clearly defining a target symptom, as well as defining the person's baseline function. Sometimes in the nursing home, the staff will use vague target symptoms. Everyone is confused about what symptom we are choosing to monitor a medication's effectiveness. If I get a call that a person is "agitated," that statement means nothing to me. I need the nurse to describe what the agitation looks like to a clear, definable target symptom. Are they hitting during care? Are they screaming "mama" for several hours? Just give me something specific to monitor. I have to grill each nurse to get specifics. But it is well worth it.

Next, get everyone on the same page. The nurse, the doctor, the resident, and the family all have to agree on the target symptom we are trying to treat. This is the ideal situation, but many times, I see conflict between staff and families about medications. Let's run through an example so you can really see how difficult the situation can become between the home and family. My nursing home had a patient name Joe. Joe was easily angered and had a fist of steel. He would box anyone who tried to change his clothes. The aides understandably did not want to be injured. They tried talking to him, explaining what they were doing, all the behavioral techniques we attempt. It was time to try a medication. The wife was not having it. She felt we wanted to medicate her husband for our own convenience. If you feel the staff is causing the agitation, there is no way you will approve medications. You basically have to show the family the baseline. Let them watch the aides getting hit. Then you can all agree on the need for treatment. The wife also did not agree her husband was confused. She felt his decisions to hit were logical, and he was defending himself. Again, we felt he was hitting due to misperceptions related to confusion. To convince a family their loved one is confused, sometimes you need to ask the memory questions in front of the family. Once we are all together, we can start a medication trial. If you are all not on the same page, it can be a disaster. It is like there are too many chefs in the pot and no agreement. The result—medications that are helping get stopped and medications that do nothing are continued. As you can see, it is a lot of stress for all. There are also times it is a more urgent situation, for example, if someone is going to attack a staff member. We do not have much time to get everyone on the same page. You may have to give the medication and explain later.

I Would Like to Be the Lipton Tea Psychiatrist

To be honest, I hate using medications. It is so freaking stressful. I wish I could just give someone a hug and some hot tea. I would be the Lipton Tea psychiatrist. No, you have to juggle multiple variables. Let's run through them quickly so you can feel how confusing it can become. You have to worry about the hitter and the people being hit. It's not just staff that is hit, it is the other residents. Of course, you have to protect the staff and the residents from injury. The family members of the victims are angry you did not protect them better. The nursing home doesn't want to be sued for injuries. Will we violate some state regulation on how we use the medications? The families maybe upset about us even considering using medications to treat the aggression. They don't believe their mom is aggressive, and we are just medicating for our convenience. What if someone gets a side effect from medications, and this makes the situation worse. Calgon, take me away. Can't we all just get along? It's a swirl of questions,

and how do you put together an answer? Then bottom line, we have to try and prevent injuries to people and maybe improve the quality of a person's life in the meantime. It's is a seemingly impossible situation to make everyone completely happy. All you and I can do is the best we can for the situation. It's never going to be perfect. I wish the drug companies would make that perfect pill with no side effects, which actually works really well. A shrink's dream come true. Nope, not happening yet. Instead we have about a handful of medications we can try to see if they help. Most have scary sounding side effects, which of course every family member has Googled and they hate. Lately, I have a bit of anxiety in my stomach each time I get a referral to see an agitated resident. I always hope I don't have to deal with all these multiple issues at one time. I just try to stick with my QQ equation each time—for my own sanity.

I do completely understand the family's frustrations. They want behavioral interventions and not medications. I wish it were always possible, but I can't control staff personally, and neither can you. There are so many unknown variables. Maybe the staff member is just not well trained, or maybe they are fully trained and your Mom is just really tough. Maybe the nurses are grumpy that day and do get snappy—they are human. Either way, you still have to make a decision in the moment about medications. You have to be prepared for that phone call from a nurse that your mom is agitated. I suppose these situations are similar to when you send your children to school. I know my daughter tried a few schools before we were happy with one. Trust me, there were days I wanted to take off a few teachers' heads. My daughter was even bit once in school when she was in 7th grade. You know bad things are going to happen, it is the price you pay for public education. You are somewhat trapped, as there is no way you can home school your child unless you're independently wealthy. You may even get a call from a teacher suggesting medication for your child. You can easily get caught up in the stress. I know it's hard to take care of the love nuggets. It's really hard. I was horrible at handling the stress when I initially started the job. I realized that getting upset at all the bad care I saw was going to kill me. I had to rework how I viewed the situation to survive. I had to work with homes that were receptive to my concerns—homes that were not perfect, but they at least they were willing to try. I can't tell you how many homes I have dropped over the years. You would think I did not need to work. It came to the point that if I personally had a parent in a home I disliked, I would rather put them through the stress of leaving this home than stay in one I hated. All I ask for is flexibility, understanding, and open-mindedness, not perfection.

So let's imagine you do get a call that a nurse would like to start medications for aggressive behaviors. I encourage you to do some investigating. Go talk to the aides that deal with your mother. Visit at night if you are told this is when Mom is the worst. See the situation from the viewpoint of the staff prior to canning the idea. If you agree, then great! The problem is solved! If you still feel she does not need medications, then make your case to the staff. Be willing to reconsider your decision if the behaviors continue. I have some families also threaten to call the lawyers if we consider medications. Lawyer talk shuts down any communication. I understand why people get to that point, but it doesn't help. I even have families bring in cameras for pictures. Nothing creates a chance to ruin good communication than taking pictures to later use in a lawsuit. I am hoping families do not see us as the enemy and go to such extremes.

If there are injuries related to you parent's behavior, then you will be pressured to start medications. Homes can feel forced into a corner at that point. They may even tell you they can no longer care for your mother safely without medications. They can send them to the psychiatric hospital under a commitment or issues them a thirty-day notice to vacate. We have to protect all the other residents. I hate to say this, but some families do not show concern when other residents are injured by their parents. This is not every family, but it is disheartening when it happens. I much prefer the family who tells me to do what I have to do to keep others safe. Regardless, it is always better to try the medication instead of forcing someone to leave a place. If the medications are not helping, it is fine to ask for a change. At least allow a period of reasonable time before you stop the trial. I have seen some families claim immediate side effects before we even tried the medication. Sometimes the family claims of side effects that cannot possibly be due to that medication—in order to sabotage the medication. I just plead for people to keep an open mind. I felt horrible recently when a woman who was seriously hallucinating and frightened was denied treatment by her niece. Her niece was basically fearful of medications. She finally agreed to let me try the medications after several lengthy conversations. Then she demanded I stop the medications within a week's time, saying the medication itself caused her to hallucinate. This was even though we all agreed she had the hallucinations before we even started the medications. I still feel bad when I walk by her aunt and watch her hallucinate.

I feel like somehow I let her down and was not able to help her mental suffering. My hands were tied.

Patient: What Is It? Me: It's an Antidepressant

Okay, now let's go to the next group of medications we have in our arsenal. I need more happy talk here! Sorry, just talking about those conflicts makes me want an antidepressant. I love my antidepressants. They, sadly, seem to be so stigmatized by society as being bad for you. People actually seem to feel more comfortable being on Xanax and Ativan instead. I hear, "Oh no, you are not putting me on those meds. They make people kill themselves." Yet the same person feels Xanax is a medical medication that is safer. If only the drug companies would change their names for these medications from *antidepressants* to *antianxiety* medications. That might help minimize the stigma. Antidepressants are really amazing medications for anxiety, not just depression. They treat all major anxiety disorders. So this is how my conversation may go with people. Patient: Can I have something for anxiety? Me: Yes, I have a great medication that will help your anxiety and it is not even addictive! Patient: What is it? Me: It's an antidepressant. Patient: "Those are for depression, and I am not even depressed." Me: "They help anxiety from panic attacks to obsessions to just excessive worry." As you can guess, I feel I have to be a saleswoman to keep people off Ativan. I am trying so hard not to be that doctor who gives everyone a tranquilizer and then gets them hooked. The pill epidemic is killing Americans daily. You really would be amazed how hard it is to get people to see antidepressant medications differently.

Early in my training, I personally was dealing with a terrible social anxiety (shyness). My doctor suggested I take Prozac. I took it really hard—to hear that suggestion. Oh my Lord, this means I am weak person. I need a crutch to be "normal," I thought. Then he said, "I just want you to experience how other people feel who are less anxious." Then I was like, "Okay, cool, if you put it that way." Wow, that stuff worked. It also helped my premenstrual crankiness (PMS), the curse to all women. A life with less shyness (and PMS) was a great relief.

Do these medications work for everyone? Heck no. They are effective about 60 percent of the time, if you are taking them properly. So if you see your Grandma crying and sad all day, why not try to see if she will fall in that number. Somehow, by boosting the brain serotonin or norepinephrine, they help. There are some that only boost serotonin: Zoloft, Lexapro, Celexa, Paxil, Prozac. Some that boost both norepinephrine and serotonin: Effexor, Cymbalta, Pristiq, Remeron. I can't go over every one of them. I can tell you one of my favorites is Remeron. That pill makes you so hungry, it's great for the elderly patients with no appetite and who are depressed. Another bonus, antidepressants also decrease anger. They figured this out when they did a study on violent criminals and realized they had low brain serotonin levels. This is very important for me as I treat a great deal of aggressive dementia residents. I love using antidepressants for aggression. Sometimes they take the edge off the anger. I especially like them for the grumpy-old-man syndrome. Trust me, many wives have also thanked me for fixing their grumpy husbands.

Now they do not want to get rid of them! Lexapro has saved several marriages I am sure.

Let's talk about side effects. Damn, they were sounding so perfect. Yes, you can get sexual side effects with some. These medications can not only lower sex drive but also make it harder to have an orgasm. For young people, this can be an advantage. Say if you are, "producing the juice before you put it in the caboose." Yes, the dreaded premature ejaculation. Antidepressants can actually lengthen that time and resolve the issue. Most elderly do not complain too much about that particular side effect in the nursing homes. When I mention it to people, many women have let me know they lost their sex drive years ago. They would rather feel less depressed than have sex. Not all antidepressants have this effect but it should be monitored. Most love nuggets are more interested is the other side effects such as dry mouth, mild constipation, night sweats—too many to list here. Some will notice these side effects before you notice any benefit. The biggest challenge is to get people past the side-effect periods. We all need to wait three to four weeks for some effect and six to eight weeks for full effect. Sometimes it takes longer in the elderly. If you can make it past the first two weeks, you probably will tolerate the medication well.

One last bit of advice about these medications. Again, make sure you have a clear target symptom you are treating. If the medication does not get rid of the target symptom at its ideal dose, then the medication has to go. You can always try a new one. Too often, people are stuck on the same medication year after year. They have lost sight of what they are trying to treat. There are times no one can tell me if the medications are helping or not. They have been taking them for years without question. Then every other doctor they see is adding other medications. I get them in the nursing home on ten to thirteen or more medications—and we are all confused. This is the good thing about nursing homes. We are required to consider tapering off the medications. If the taper fails, they stay on the medications.

I obviously can't fix every person's depression with pills, but I will try as hard as I can for them, especially if the depression is really lowering the quality of life for a person. I think dementia with depression is more challenging. I personally find that such patients have trouble responding to the medications. I wonder if some of this has to do with poor coping skills due to frontal lobe issues. I also wonder how much the neurotransmitters are damaged and the medications cannot increase them as easily.

Antipsychotics

Next is the third group of pills—the hardest to explain. They are the antipsychotics. These medications try to reverse psychosis. They actually do it by lowering a neurotransmitter called dopamine. They are the medications such as Haldol, Risperdal, Seroquel, Abilify, Zyprexa, and Geodon. As I have said, paranoia is a psychotic symptom that is a big trigger for violence. This is why these medications are sometimes chosen for the more aggressive residents. Actually, we try to reserve them specifically for aggression only for reasons I will elaborate.

Delirium

My first real experience prescribing an antipsychotic was in medical school. We were all geeky medical students in our new white coats. We had a bunch of reference guides packed in our pockets to look up "stuff" we did not know. We were like the psych swat team of the hospital. We were called one day to see a belligerent older guy ready to take out our staff. I was all big eyed and scared, waiting to see what my teacher would do next to control him. He says, "Haldol 10 mg and if it does not work in an hour, then 20 mg." It was called rapid sedation. I was thinking, "Wow, that's a lot of drugs." We thumbed through our books to see if he was correct, and rapid sedation was a real thing. My teacher was a bit eccentric so we didn't know what to believe. But, he knew what he was saying. By the time this guy had his second dose of Haldol, he was purring like a kitten. Meow, meow. He was holding a normal conversation and fully alert. Our teacher was always telling us, "Antipsychotics organize people." I will never forget this as I have repeatedly seen it again and again. He then went on to say that tranquilizers could make people possibly more disorganized and confused. He preferred antipsychotics for confused aggression to tranquilizers.

This guy in the hospital was suffering from what we call a "delirium." I still work in the medical hospital and have seen hundreds of delirious patients since that day. Delirium is basically confusion related to an acute medical condition. It is not the same as dementia. Delirium can be reversible and dementia is not. The actual definition of delirium is a waxing and waning of consciousness. One minute they can be alert and coherent, the next they are sleepy and confused. This is why we tend to avoid the tranquilizers with delirium as these medications can increase confusion. The other main symptoms of delirium are hallucinations, paranoia, and disorientation. While someone is in a delirium, they can also present as dangerous to themselves and others. My job is to make sure the patient doesn't rip out all their IV lines and tubes as the medical staff is trying to figure out the medical reasons for the delirium. We have two ways to keep their agitation from delirium controlled in the hospital—medications and physical restraints. I hate seeing people tied to beds, as it can make them more agitated. Then again, it is kind of scary when you see an older guy pull a catheter out his bladder. They don't realize that at the end of the tube that is going into their bladder, there is a little balloon blown up. So when they pull it, it takes the balloon across the prostate and can tear up the pathway for the urine. I am sure that made every male reader cringe. How the heck do people really do this? They are so confused they do not even realize what they are doing. A nursing home obviously would not be able to handle this same person. They are not allowed to retrain at all. Nursing homes are always returning people to the hospital after a tube was pulled. People can even pull the feeding tubes out of their stomachs. We have also had several people pull the breathing tubes out of their necks in confusion. They touch it and think, what is this doing here? The next thing they can't breathe as they are waving around the breathing tube in the air. This is obviously when restraints come into play.

Physical Restraints

People frequently ask why we can't restrain in nursing homes? Pretty simple—it is against the regulations. I assume it's from years when nursing homes were getting away with abuses, that the state inspectors took away all our tools. Many families still ask us to physically restrain their families to prevent injury. I do not think they are trying to be mean, they are really trying to help us prevent injury. Say for instance, we are trying to stop people from falling. We can't sit next to them all day to prevent a fall. Because we can't restrain, people have developed a few tricks of the trade I have noticed. For the weak, unsteady person who insists they can walk, the nurses push their wheelchair under a dining room table and lock the chair wheels. It does not look like a restraint, just that you are sitting at a table. You can also put the restless fallers in a very low bed and surround it with floor mats. It is really hard for an eighty year old to stand up when they are so low to the ground. Lastly, there is the annoying chair alarm. Every time the unsteady person tries to stand, it will go off. They can be fairly easily disconnected when they end up annoying the heck out of someone. I think these alarms make us feel better we're trying to prevent falls. I have seen many nurses do fifty-yard dashes toward a wheelchair when the alarm goes off, only to be a second too late. As patients are getting discharged faster and faster from the hospital, and sicker and sicker, we have to be more creative. If this sounds like an impossible situation, it pretty much is one. People are going to keep falling.

Chemical Restraints

Besides the physical restraints, we have chemical restraints. The situation is again different between the hospitals and the nursing homes. In hospitals, we can use Haldol. Remember? The rapid sedation medication. We try to get rid of all the Haldol before the nursing homes come to take them. The nursing homes are afraid to use Haldol as, for a period, it was overused and the state frowns on it the most. It also has long-term side effects, and it really should only be used short term. We go more for Risperdal and Seroquel in the homes. Either way, we need a medication to help to control this severe type of agitation. In the hospital where I now work, I am asked several times a week to help get the patients calmer with medications so they can remove the wrist restraints. If we are not able to remove the restraints, the person is stuck in the hospital. A nursing home rehab will not look at them with the restraints. Once they are calmer, the hospital calls several nursing homes to "review" the situation. Many will decline the agitated to avoid the risks. Some have a low census and need the money: they may accept the patient.

Let me break from antipsychotics to discuss one more issue in regards to delirium. Delirium is a very serious and scary syndrome. Why? Once you develop it, you may never be the same again. This is probably one of the most important points in this book. If an elderly person develops delirium, say after a surgery, it is not a good prognostic sign. Of those elderly developing delirium, approximately 40 percent will die the following year. One-third may remain confused after the surgery for up to six months. Another 30 percent will develop some degree of dementia. Medicare spends 100 billion in costs related to delirium. This is why doctors themselves will refuse surgery later in life. Many surgeons do not emphasize this risk prior to surgery. So when someone goes in for an elective heart or orthopedic surgery, this has to be taken into account. If someone is advanced in age (over eighty), has any degree of dementia, or several serious medical issues before surgery, you will be at higher risk of developing delirium after surgery. You have to be willing to take the risk of never coming out the same after surgery. In the best-case scenario, the delirium will fully resolve and you can go home. Then there are those who are not resolving and will need nursing home care. Many end up in the homes just to "let them clear up." They may never fully clear. Please just take this into account before you agree to any major surgery.

Delirium is not always after surgery, and not just in the hospitals. I also have delirium develop in people who are long-term residents of the nursing homes. For example, we have a woman named Agnes in one of our homes. She does have dementia as her baseline. Every now and then, we see Agnes getting angry and paranoid. We all know what is up. Agnes has another bladder infection. She has developed a mild delirium from infection. I have no idea why the brain is so connected to the bladder. We would joke in training that we used more antibiotics to help out agitated elderly than psychiatric drugs. If the antibiotic did not clear up her anger, she would get a few weeks of Seroquel. Works like a charm.

Something happened in the last five years that really shook up the nursing homes' use of antipsychotics. A big study was a released discussing the dangers of antipsychotics in the elderly. This study caused us all to have to rethink everything. It was already tough that we have only a few choices with medications. Then they have to do some research and make life more complicated. It is not that I want people getting side effects; I am just running out of ideas on what we can use to help. Basically, they did a large study that showed elderly who were given antipsychotics for dementia related behavioral disorders have a 1.6–1.7 times increased risk of death. Most deaths were related to heart disease or infections like pneumonia. Well, then the witch hunt began. Medicare is all over these medications now. Inspectors are scouring the charts of the people on them. "Why did you start this medication? Why can't you stop it?" "Why didn't you try alternatives?" I have even recently heard these drugs are "abusive". As I have learned in life, not everything is all good or all bad. These medications control violence so that many can stay at home and out of nursing homes. Behaviors are a big trigger to nursing home placement. I would never try to make a family feel bad for needing to rely on these medications.

We all know we need to try to avoid them and I pride myself on getting people off of them over time. I do not need a law or rule to get me to try reductions of all these medications. I had been doing it already. If we reduce the drugs and the person starts to beat up people again, then the drug taper can be called unsuccessful. The state then feels the use of the medications are fine at that point. The next six months to a year, we consider another taper. This new study has just added a whole new layer of stress to that phone call I receive after a person has been violent. I am dreading having to use chemical restraints. What medication do I give now? How do I tell a family the medication I use can kill their Mom? I can give Ativan but we already said that is not a great alternative. I can try a happy pill that takes weeks to work. At what point do you say we have to use the antipsychotic or someone will be injured. So, if you are wondering why many doctors do not want my job, I am thinking it is fairly clear now. Let's just say there is a big shortage of psychiatrists in nursing homes.

All we can do is what I have said many times—monitor medications closely. Only use antipsychotics if someone is a danger to themselves or others, or their paranoia is so severe that it is ruining the quality of their lives. So, I guess it goes back to my Q/Q equation again. If someone is dying and they are seeing scary hallucinations, you can bet your left big toe I am giving them Seroquel. I am not concerned it will make them sleepy or give them a heart attack, as it is less of an evil as mental or physical suffering.

Antipsychotic Side Effects

If these medications are monitored properly by people who understand their risks, they are a powerful tool. You will always get different opinions on which is the best, but I feel comfortable with

Seroquel. I will tell you why. It is generally void of one specific side effect that drives me crazy, "drug-induced Parkinsonism." It is not Parkinson's disease, but you look as if you have Parkinson's. It is also called pseudo or false Parkinson's. Other antipsychotics such as Risperdal, when used over time, can cause these Parkinson's-like effects. It is a bad consequence of blocking the dopamine in your brain. Dopamine is the neurotransmitter that is involved in how your body moves. So if you block it in your brain, then your body may move incorrectly. You will start to shuffle in your gait, your arms will swing less when you walk, you will start to stoop over. Your arms will stiffen and you may even notice a hand tremor. It can even stiffen your swallowing and lead to aspiration and pneumonias. Risperdal slows the swallowing mechanism for some. Seroquel has the lowest risk of the Parkinson's side effect. Seroquel is not a perfect medication, but it at least doesn't cause this mess.

Of course, many doctors do not monitor for the stiffness. I have had countless elderly admitted to nursing homes from the community after developing Parkinsonism. The doctors leave the Risperdal for months until the person stiffens and keeps falling. It is a hard side effect to reverse. You really have to be aware of it, and I am telling my nurses to watch for it. This is again why it is positive we are always trying to reduce and eliminate these medications. As in any situation, we have to weigh the pros and cons and make the best choice.

Seizure Medications

There is one last medication option. It is not a mind blowing one. It is the seizure medications. I have not been as impressed with them, but they are always available. Medications such as Trileptal and Depakote. Remember when I spoke about the frontal lobe, and how damage to it can cause people to be impulsive? I tend to use these medications on this category of people. Sexually or physically impulsive people can be good candidates. They sometimes help.

Other Medications

There are other medications the drug companies would really want you to choose. They are the Alzheimer's medications like Aricept and Exelon. They are marketed to delay the progression of the illness, or delay nursing home placement, or delay the length of time someone will develop severe dementia. They are fine when someone is at home early in the disease, but I see more people already advanced and past these markers. I do not generally use these medications. When the FDA study came out blasting antipsychotics, the Aricept/Exelon people were advocating that their medications also helped the behaviors of dementia. They were hoping Aricept would replace the other medications to treat behaviors. They even have some studies to back it up. I personally have not seen them help. Of course, I deal with really agitated people and we can't wait for the chance Aricept may or may not work. We may be waiting forever, and someone will get hurt. The other concern I have about them is that they may drop your heart rate. You will see people start to pass out as they develop the low heart rates. I have seen people end up with pacemakers on these drugs. The doctors do not always seem to be aware of this side effect. I just want people to know these medications have risks. They seem to be more acceptable to people, as they are not considered psychiatric medications. I really do not even consider them a fifth option.

Well, this is my brief synopsis on medications. It was not the purpose of this book to go over them in great detail. Just a rough and dirty guide. To summarize, we can choose a between tranquilizers, antidepressants, antipsychotics, or seizure medications. Each group has several options under it. They are only different in some side effects or cost. You can ask your doctor to choose which they like the best. I only try to use them once we have ruled out medical illnesses for the psychiatric issue or if behavioral techniques do not help.

I do not want you all to think every decision to start these medications result in a great deal of conflict. Most of the time, it goes very smoothly, and families are very agreeable. I just want you all to be mentally prepared for the worst. This is the bread-and-butter of my job and really hard to explain all these issues in the ten minutes I have at the bedside. I am assuming after all this explanation, you all understand now why I think Grandma may do better with marijuana. People would be so relaxed and not fighting. There would be no issues with loss of appetite. It may cost the home more money in munchie availability. Okay, maybe instead of smoking it, we should just make the magic marijuana brownies available. We don't need to start any fires.

CHAPTER 6

A Typical Day

Now you all know pretty much what I know after years dealing with dementia and nursing homes. People were interested in what a typical day is like for me, so I threw this chapter in here. I will be totally honest about what nursing homes ask me to do, no matter how unbelievable. There are days I wonder if what is happening is real, or a strange part of my imagination. What I mean will be self-evident as you read along. I wish I could add humor to it all, but sometimes even I am at a loss. A typical day starts with the nurses reporting to me all the tough situations they are trying to resolve. I go in, get my list, and try to pin them all down on exactly what they are looking for me to do. If it sounds impossible, I tell them up front. For example, I can't stop people who are smearing feces. They are removed from the list. Oddly enough, the day I wrote this chapter was an involuntary commitment day. I was asked to do what is called a Baker Act. A Baker Act is the Florida word for an involuntary commitment for anyone who is a potential danger to self or others. I was called when an elderly male named Fred was becoming very assaultive toward his peers. Fortunately for me, one of the nurse practitioners in the home had already completed the Baker Act forms. I sighed a bit of relief that I would not be the one to take the heat from the family for sending him to the hospital—so I thought.

Fred, the Ticking Time Bomb

Let me tell you about Fred. I had been working with Fred for a few years. He had a bad temper and we were always a little nervous around him. I was always able to keep him from getting too violent. We never knew what would set him off. He then started to become more territorial around his room. He would start to threaten his roommates as if they did not belong on his property. He had tried to pull one peer from the bed whom he felt was an imposter. I told the home to not let him have a roommate for fear he would harm the person. They did not take my advice: what can I do? I felt bad for the roommate. Imagine being in your bed as you feel a hand grab your arm. Then a strong pull as you find yourself falling on the floor. I imagine this is what it would feel like for the other guy. Fred was a ticking time bomb.

Several times prior to this episode, I had tried different medication changes on him to prevent him from ending up in a hospital. The hospital is always the worst possible outcome. It does, however, allow us to change the medications under a safe setting for all involved. Let me ask you, if you were me, how many chances would you give Fred before you sent him to a hospital? Who is going to watch him every second to be sure he doesn't hurt someone else? What do you say to the family of the person he hurt! Today was different. Fred had finally gone too far, and enough was enough. He now was randomly targeting residents in wheelchairs. He was trying to pull them out of chairs. He was feeling everyone was an intruder and they all had to leave. He was even firing the nursing staff. By the time I got there, the staff had shot him with a dose of Ativan. He had calmed enough to speak to his son who had arrived by then and was talking to him. The son let me know that his father, still calm from Ativan, felt bad for his behavior and was apologetic. Of course, I was waiting for the request to drop the Baker Act, as Fred was sorry. It really was not anything I could change at that point: he was officially committed by the ARNP. This is the tricky part of dementia, I explained to the son. The patient may have a rapidly shifting frame of reference every hour. He will totally forget the entire situation in a few hours and would be back to the same old guy. I would love to go home, say no harm no foul, and have the son sing my praises. Life would be so much easier. Fred had crossed the line this time going after so many residents. Everyone was too frightened.

I reminded the son that his dad was on edge constantly. I was always afraid to ask his father anything. He was the perfect example of walking on eggshells. He answered a lot of questions with, "what do you mean." This is a dangerous expression and warning sign for me that someone is paranoid. For instance, after he pulled his roommate out of the bed, I asked Fred if he would be accepting of a new man in his room. This is when he pulled out the "what do you mean" line. Of course you want to say, "what do you mean, what do I mean?" The "what do you mean" is a sign for you to slowly back out of the room with a pleasant smile. If you change the subject fast and act stupid, that works well also. It's typical of a chronically paranoid person who is not processing information well to act this way. I was not surprised when I received the call he had been Baker Acted. I assume another innocent peer said something to set him off, not realizing he was a ticking time bomb. Sadly, we have no control of what another confused person could say to him.

I had a long and stressful conversation with his son, who was still not fully accepting that his father even had dementia at all. He felt his father was in full control of his behavior. An apology should be enough to end the issue in his mind. If a doctor and family are on different pages as to the diagnosis, it is as if we are speaking different languages. I tried to explain dementia again—still not working. The son then repeated the same observation at least four times. "He probably just has a urinary tract infection, he always is bad when he has those." I would agree if his father were not always having temper issues. He was worse with bladder infections, but the staff informed me that was not the case. He had no significant bladder infection that day.

As I have said, I do understand the tendency to defend a family member and not accept they are dangerous. However, Fred almost took out two or three other peers. Thank goodness staff was there to stop him. What if an innocent bystander was injured? I can't look at what is best for Fred and Fred alone. I have to look at all the people who will potentially be harmed. This son could not expand his focus beyond his anger at the situation. So what was the cure? There are no real cures. There is only doing your best until the dementia process progresses past the aggressive stage. I wish I had a better answer. I wish there was a behavioral technique I could do to calm him, but once a person hits the peaks of paranoia, not much works besides a medication. He eventually went to the hospital and later transferred to a new home. I hate to say it, but if a family is not able to see the full seriousness of the aggression, then the relationship with the home can be damaged. The home wants a family to acknowledge the concern others may be injured by their loved ones behavior. At that point a new start maybe the best option. As you can see, there really is no worse situation than having to Baker Act someone. It is, and always will be, a last resort.

Charlotte and the Crying

The next lady on the list, named Charlotte, I was asked to see was for crying. I had been trying to get her to stop crying for months. She was a frail skinny woman who never left her bed. She spoke with a British accent when she did choose to speak. She would cry and when asked why she cried, would never answer why. She would also frequently hallucinate and talk to people who were not there. Of course, it was not happy conversations. Today, she told me someone in her family told a lie that she was dead. I knew arguing with her delusion would go nowhere. I generally will try one time to redirect. "Why would someone say you are dead—maybe it was a misunderstanding?" She cried and insisted I was wrong. I gave it a shot to change her mind. It failed in seconds, so I went off to increase the paranoia medications. The nurses had even tried to talk her out of her paranoia as well. She was mentally so uncomfortable. She now has moments of calmness with medication, but I have not been able to take the delusions completely away.

Edith Didn't Yell This Time

Down the hallway was a 92-year-old female pistol named Edith. I asked them to stop putting her on my list as she drove me a little insane. I knew I couldn't really fix her anyways. I would just sit and listen to her talk, as she really didn't care what I said. If I just sat and nodded, she loved me. She would say, "Come again anytime." I would just be thinking, "Thank God that's over with. She didn't yell at me and invited back even." She would sometimes yell at me just because I was a psychiatrist, and it must mean someone thinks she is "crazy" if I was sent to see her. She would also tell me she thought the social worker was having sex with some man in her bathroom. She rationalized that was okay as it is "a normal thing for young people." I'm not sure why she would think anyone would choose to have sex in her bathroom. I am sure there are several other more ideal locations to procreate for a young person. She also felt the charge nurse had it out for her. She would visit the director of nurses daily with her proof of the abuse. The medications really did not put a dent in her paranoia. They stopped only the worst of her agitation, the physical part. She would try to physically attack the nurses, and the meds did help this symptom. I try to be honest what I can and cannot fix with medications. She has adjusted to the point of no longer needing the medications, but still a bit of a conspiracy creator.

George: "Nice Tush!"

In the same hall was the flirty guy named George. I was asked several times to see him to get him to stop making sexual comments to staff. He would basically ask them for sex. I tried talking to him once. I told him the nurses did not appreciate the cuteness of their derrieres discussed. I asked him to stop kindly. He of course denied it and laughed me off. I kept telling the nurses to ignore his comments. I can't stop flirtation. To be honest, I feel the nurses should be flattered at the compliments. It's when they stop commenting on your tush that you should worry. All kidding aside, I don't get concerned until they go after the other residents. Thankfully, most will go after the young and firm versus the old and saggy. Problem solved.

Donald with the Greasy Hair

Down to the locked dementia unit, the one unit that has the most battle stories. There is a large glass window where we can watch them all walk by us. Many a confused nugget will tap on it and try to have a logical conversation with us. There is one guy named Donald who will tap, wave, and smile repeatedly. You have to stop what you are doing to wave at least four or five times. You don't want to be rude and ignore him. He is so hard to bathe in the shower that his hair starts to grow down his neck in a long greasy fashion. I was asked several times to see him in hopes I could help him be more compliant with bathing. Each time we asked him to bathe, he would argue that he already had a shower today. I finally was so sick of looking at his hair one day, I found an aide with some scissors. I flirted with him until we cut off the length. It was a temporary high of success. As you know, hair grows back. He was there again today, still had long greasy hair. Oh well, another fail for my medications. Back to the female charms again.

I usually will walk the halls of the dementia unit and just check out situations. I can't do therapy with them, as they are too confused. There is always at least one person screaming, sometimes you will hear another resident say "Shut Up!" There are a few pacers, every now and then setting off the exit alarms. They will walk non-stop like they have motors. I have the one Latina who dances and laughs. You think she is always happy until someone pisses her off, then you can see the Cuban side come out. I can only say this for sure as I married a Cuban.

Carol: The Zoloft Worked!

I ran into my tough patient named Carol finally. She was so angry to be there when she first moved in the place. She was constantly telling me she was tired of being held against her will for no reason. Today, she told me she was content. The Zoloft worked! It restored my faith in medications.

Havoc-Causing Elsie

Sometimes the aides will approach me to tell me their issues with the residents. "She just bent back my hand," I hear in passing. Oh no, they were talking about a 97-year-old named Elsie, still strong enough to cause havoc. It is at times hard to believe what the aides were saying about Elsie. The aide even recreated for me how she twisted her arm back. Then you look at Elsie and think it has to be impossible. This lady looked 90 pounds soaking wet. She was so deaf that that is was hard to ask her about what happened. I tried several times to find out and all she would say is, "can you take me to the bathroom?" "Yes ma'am, I'll get someone." I left with my tail between my legs. I was not going to drug up a 97-year-old. I took the easy way out; I assumed she had another bladder infection so we ordered up another test.

Cranky George

The next guy was George, an 89-year-old man who was there just for physical therapy after a hip fracture. I was seeing him, as he was not eating well and refusing to get out of bed. He was a really cranky guy. He let me know he lived with his daughter, and he felt she was a "terrible caregiver." I sighed in relief she was not there at the time to hear him. He let me know he was in too much pain to sit in a wheelchair; he had too much pressure on the hip. He let me know he did not care if he lived or died. He was skinny as a beanpole and made no eye contact. I always try to meet people where they are at in the moment, no arguments from me. I tell them it's fine if they want to give up, I get it. I let them vent. Most families would cringe because I don't really argue. If you argue, then you are not validating how they feel. The best way to know if they are serious is to take it to the next level. I tell them how they will probably need to give up independent living if they are quitting therapy. Sometimes, they think about what giving up means, and then they change their minds. This guy clearly was ready to quit. His body was exhausted and he was going to make himself comfortable. You can generally see the long-term people coming. I started him on an antidepressant; we will see if it changes his mind.

Mildred Was Really Ill

The next woman, Margaret, had refused to see me several times. I was used to walking in and then walking right back out. I even banned the staff from putting her on my list. Of course, no matter how hard I tried, they kept asking me to see her. She did not like psychiatrists. Maybe it was because her husband, Sam, had had severe bipolar disorder for several years. She was probably grouping us all in the "psychiatrist's-just-drug-people-up" category. I knew her husband well before he died. Even when I would visit him, Margaret would never try to interact with me. When he finally did die, the nurses thought for sure she was seriously depressed. They had been a lively couple, and she was just not the same any longer. They convinced me to try to see her again, and in no time, she kicked me out again. What's a shrink to do? Take her off the list again please!

I finally had one more call to see her; this was a persistent nursing staff. She had become much more confused and was hallucinating today. She was refusing to sleep in her room and was now sleeping in a wheelchair. I told them, sounds medical and not psych. The medical people started an antidepressant despite my feelings. People sometimes confuse medical weakness with depression. The family then had the antidepressant stopped and then blamed her confusion on the antidepressant of course. I get this a lot. It's never the medical medications causing the problem, always the psychiatric ones. Well, she was still confused even off the Paxil. Then the medical people finally wanted her to go to the ER for the confusion, but the family declined. They all again blamed the psych meds for causing prolonged confusion even after the medication was stopped. The nurses badgered me to go back in to see her, I gave in. I was sure she would kick me out again, but maybe with her confusions she would forget I was a psychiatrist? I had a few theories of what was going on before I even entered the room. She was afraid to sleep in her room: maybe she was paranoid? She didn't want to lie flat in the bed: maybe another case of congestive heart failure? I was ready to problem solve.

She was in her wheelchair, wearing oxygen. She was not the strong woman whose eyes would pierce in anger the last few times. I knew right away she was not well. She did what all really ill people do; they fall asleep while they are speaking in mid-sentence. Her hands were cool and her pulse felt up. I asked her about paranoia and she denied feeling this way. I asked her if she had seen her deceased husband. It's always a sign someone is ready to go. She of course thought I was nuts, "He is dead of course." Well, she passed that test. I asked how much she thought about him. "I think about him all night long," she said. She did not say what the thoughts were, but it touched my heart. She was also not the worst delirium I had ever seen but still looked quite ill. I then went to the nurse, and I told her she needed to go to the ER. She reminded me that the family had declined the transfer earlier in the week. I felt pretty confident this was serious and convinced them to listen to me. They agreed to send her out. I waited a week to find out what happened. Margaret finally passed to heaven due to a pulmonary embolism. I did not expect that fully, but I was glad she was with her husband. The nurses later told me the family was there looking for their father's ashes. Apparently, Margaret had left them in her clothes drawer. Now, they were unable to locate them. This situation went from bad to worse. I can't help but having that awful thought that his ashes ended up in the same spot as where all the lost dentures end up. All I know is that Margaret and Sam are together again— that's the most important thing.

Ornery Ben

Ben was next on my list. I actually loved Ben. I was asked to see him because he was so upset by his own behaviors. He was being so mean to people for no reasons. I love the ornery guys who not only say rude things, but can also laugh about it at the same time. He was hard to find in the building at first as he was always at AA meetings. I am not sure how he did it, but he was able to get there in his wheelchair. He was a hardcore alcoholic, who had been sober for thirty years. His whole life was built around sobriety. Within minutes of meeting him, he let me know he had just fired his doctor for not writing an order he needed fast enough. He also let me know he was upset at himself for being mean. I was a bit surprised he was feeling so guilty. He had a reputation around the home for being mean, not a reputation for being remorseful. This was the same guy who told a 90-year-old demented woman the meanest thing I ever heard. She was Jewish and had survived the concentration camps. She would cry loudly everyday for her "people." One day he yelled at her, "wish we could send you back to the concentration camps." I know, pretty mean. So needless to say, he was a real bastard. So, I listened some more to his story. He was happy I knew a lot about AA as I had been working with young addicts lately. I even offered for him to come speak at one of the AA meetings at my work. I know that the young addicts would believe him more than I about the dangers of drinking. He let me know something that completely surprised me—that he was too embarrassed for people to see him. He showed me his legs, they were thin and bruised. He started to wear arm covers to hide his thinning skin. He told me how depressed he was feeling and how little he really was thinking of himself. He had felt guilt over firing his doctor. Someone so tough, weakened by the years of aging. I promised him I would start an antidepressant and come check on him again. His story reminded me of how we can build our self-image around our body's appearance. Seems like a dangerous place to rest your self-esteem since we all are going to lose our youthful appearances.

Sam Scares Us All

The last person on the list today was Sam. He has dementia, although we couldn't convince his wife of this fact. He would grab remote controls and threaten to kill the nurses, with a stabbing motion of course. His wife would say, "Stop that Sam, they are going to think you are crazy." Of course, she didn't know that is exactly what we thought. He was a strong guy and could do damage. He eventually went to the hospital and we were all afraid to take him back. We were not afraid so much of the patient, we were afraid of the wife. She didn't get that his behaviors were from dementia. She didn't get that no one wanted to take care of him for fear of an injury. So somehow we had to convince her to let us start some medication to help prevent injuries. I told the nurses there was no way I was starting any medications until she was on board. I am not sure how they did it, but she finally agreed to give him something. I am pretty sure they told her that without medications they were not going to be able to care for him. So far, he is somewhat more manageable.

Joyce, the Wife

I see another woman, Joyce, in the homes weekly. She's not a patient, she is actually a wife. Her husband I have seen for years because he was always so combative. He makes these odd yells at times and shakes his whole body. He finally stopped trying to hit staff. She sits with him daily, she is always there. She talks with him at times, then she will ask me about his medications to control his anger—curious to see what dose he is on and if it needs to be raised or lowered. I see her exhausted body and over the weeks, her hair appears more greasy and thin. I feel like the situation is aging her. Her husband so loud and full of life, as if he were taking hers. I have told her to stop coming in so much, to care for herself. She never listens. She wants to be there for him, quietly, with no fanfare or thanks. I wish I could infuse her with life again. I get her mission, I watch her from afar hoping one day her stress is over.

The Forgotten Aids

The nursing homes are just not the patients and the families. They are the forgotten aides. I pass the same ones weekly. I always wonder who hurt them today. I feel horrible over what I know they go through. The number of times they are called racial slurs. I see one in particular who says "hello" back to me. Many are shy, reserved Haitian or Jamaican women. I always ask her who is beating her up today, and I will go take care of them. She gives me a room number. Lately, it has been a guy named John. He throws his dirty Depends on the floor and then tells her that it is her job to pick it up. Of course, John blames the aides for his behavior. He feels they provoked him into being cruel. I hate to see anyone being treated badly. I try to make sure she knows I care. I crack a stupid joke to make her laugh. I figure at least if she knows someone is bothered by the cruelty she deals with daily, it will make her job easier.

Gert the Dancer

At the end of my day at this building, a singer named Max Green always comes to perform. All the women run to see him. I have even been cut off once by a woman during an interview, letting me know our talk was over and that she had to see Max. He was a younger guy that played a mean piano. He was bearded and a little rough looking. Even as women age, they still like the tough guys. I stand there and watch the people dance. One woman named Gert is always there. She is so confused, but one hot dancer. She spins and smiles right in front of the stage as if it's a live concert. I hate to say it, but I can never tell if she has on a bra—I am sure an added bonus for all the older men in the audience. I imagine her in her younger years doing the same. The staff sometimes dances with them and it's all a lot of fun. I love that I can get a brief moment of joy in a day filled with sadness and horror at times. This makes the whole thing feel better for a moment. Thank you Gert. Thanks for making my typical day less typical.

CHAPTER 7

Letting Go: When Is Enough Going to Be Enough

➤ When to intervene?
➤ Hospice.
➤ Pain management and sedation.
➤ Decision making and guilt.
➤ Failure to thrive.
➤ Discussions of death and dying.
➤ DNR.
➤ "Skilled" Medicare benefits.

"The purpose of any doctor or any human in general should not
be to simply delay the death of the patient, but to increase the
person's quality of life."
—*Patch Adams, M.D.*

The Push and Pull of Old Age

I love Patch Adams. He believed in humor and play as essential
to emotional and physical health. I see this at our entertainment
dances in the nursing homes. One of my favorite activities now is
to do stupid dances for old people. There is nothing better than
watching them smile as I act goofy. I love to watch them dance
as well. I notice the pelvic gyrations are much different than the
hip-hop gyrations of the young. It is more of a twisting and less
of a thrusting. They don't seem to care as long as they are moving
and being silly. Despite all my horror stories about homes, it's not

always doom and gloom and people beating each other up. The way to survive at times is to cherish the silliness.

However, no matter how much I tried to wrap myself up in the fun, I still had a nagging problem. I was sick of seeing people suffer needlessly. I must say—I *did* burn out. I watched as others burned out with me. Why? We struggled with watching people decline and suffer in unnecessary ways. We struggled with unrealistic expectations people have of our medical interventions. Despite all our medical miracles, we could not stop the march of aging and physical decline. I felt a medical intervention was an opportunity and calculated risk, not a promise of health. A typical day was wearing on me and those around me.

There is a constant push and pull in all our decisions. We are trying to keep people alive, customers happy, and keep the regulators off our back. If someone loses weight, we were on it pressuring them to eat. The fall squads were trying to prevent falls. We knew we really couldn't stop all falls. We all just held our breaths that no one would break a bone. Then we had those who were frequently ill and declining. They were constantly in and out of the hospitals with no improvement. It is hard to watch the merry-go-round, especially when you see residents with no improvement in their quality of life.

When do we stop all the interventions? Well, I can tell you if we had an accepting family, the job was clear. We could start keeping them comfortable with less intervention. If we did not have a family mentally prepared for a decline, then there would be countless meetings explaining why mom is failing, adding in some finger pointing. There was pressure to do physical therapy on people we knew would never benefit, then seemingly endless medical procedures afterward. Sometimes, the actual patient was lost in the conversation. To make it worse, the patient had dementia and many times was not able to be involved in the conversation. We all made decisions for them, choices they may have never wanted to be made if they were of sound mind.

Conflict: Doctors, Nurses, Families

The nurses and the aides see every aspect of the human condition. When dealing with dementia residents in the home, each pill given, every injection, blood draw, and catheter placed, we think, "When is enough going to be enough?" I have never met a nurse who has not told me, "If I get this way, please do me in." We all joke about our large pill stash we will take when the time is ready." In reality, we are actually serious. We are there all day in homes and can't escape the reality of the human condition. I personally could never be a nurse, but I admire those who can do what they are asked. Many times, they have to follow a doctor's order whether they agree or not. I am sure we put them in awful positions as doctors. I am sure they do not want to lose their hard-earned license by disagreeing with orders we write. They are frustrated at times with us doctors just going along with every bad idea a family suggests. I have had so many nurses tell me privately they were so happy I "stood up to the family." What they really meant is they are happy I talked someone out of an unnecessary medical intervention. I did not let an angry family member sway me away from what is best for a resident. I am sad it has become an "us against them" mentality, but this is where we are heading.

Speaking of bad ideas for medical interventions, I think back to my mother's black potions and yeast-free diets. I get why she held out hope for cures that just didn't exist. I suppose if I were diagnosed with dementia, I probably would do hundreds of Google searches trying to find that perfect concoction to take for a longer life. There is that point however, where the cures start to ruin the quality of life. I feel bad for the residents in the homes who are taking lengthy "healthy" remedies of pills. Imagine taking ginkgo biloba, Namenda, fish oil, and whatever else you can find to keep your brain working. I can barely take a multivitamin without burping it up all day. If I thought there was actually a cure for dementia, I would slurp that pill down even if it tasted like beets. I think you understand my point. Nothing would stop me from taking that pill I knew would cure dementia. Since that pill does not exist, I am always trying to limit the number of pills a person has to take daily. Sometimes side effects are overlooked as we hold onto the false hopes of medications.

The H-Bomb

If we bring up the hospice word to people, that's a whole other issue. No one wanted to be the one to drop the "H-bomb." Some staff member would finally cave to say to the family, "Would you consider hospice?" Then the long pause to see how they reacted. Many families were so angry because they felt it is a sign we were giving up on the patient. I suppose it can be seen this way, but hospice seems to be very different lately. I can see why people are confused. One of the main criteria to go on hospice, is that a doctor has to say you have six months or less to live. I think this is why most people understood hospice easier if they had cancer. But many times we are dealing with dementia only. How do you know when the six-month mark starts with dementia? Once hospice is ordered, the nice hospice people come into the nursing home and start the services. You have care in place. Medicare will cover hospice services. We can then keep the patient comfortable and the family supported. The musicians, social workers, priests all come to visit to comfort you. We stop all the excessive medical procedures. It seems very straightforward, but no, anything dealing with death never is simple. As I have said, it's not so easy to predict when a person with dementia will die. What do we do then?

I remember when I asked a woman out of curiosity how she felt her hospice services were for her husband. He had recently passed away. She said, "I hated hospice, they killed my husband." **What?** I nearly fell on the floor. I knew I could not ask her what she thought hospice meant and that death was the goal. I also wondered how often hospice is accused of murder based on her comment? Apparently they were just doing their job, and they did it successfully. I knew we in the medical field are accused of murder—but *not* hospice. They are like little angels of mercy. I really thought about what she said. I suppose she must have been fearful hospice pushed him along too quickly. I was actually very happy when my mother was on the morphine drip, and maybe it did push her over that edge. I mean, morphine does technically suppress your drive to breathe. You could say they killed her faster than the cancer did? If you think about it, you could classify it as murder of a dying person? I also wonder if people panic when they see their family member getting too sleepy from pain medications. Maybe it is like a final reality check that they are dying? We want someone to be comfortable and not in pain, but also fully alert and talking to family. It is really hard to accomplish that balance. All I know is doctors do not want to be accused of *murder*, and I have seen them withhold needed pain medication if pressured. This situation is really complicated.

Terri Schiavo

I am frequently reminded of the story of Terri Schiavo and how it was considered murder to remove her feeding tube. Terri was in a persistent vegetative state and was not able to tell others what she wanted. Apparently she told her husband before her illness that she did not want to be kept alive if she had no chance of recovery. Her parents did not believe the doctors about her medical condition, and wanted her feeding tube left in, hoping her brain would heal. This caught national attention including involvement from President George W. Bush and his brother Jeb Bush, Governor of Florida. What people do not know is that issues like this come up everyday with no fanfare—the question of when to let someone go. We are all stuck with figuring this dilemma out without courts or presidents intervening. I think families hold out hope that a miracle will happen. As with Terri's parents, they were waiting for her brain to return. We all have spoken to that distant family member, or that person who Googled, "The doctors told them they were going to die, and the next thing you know they are up talking." The wait for the miracle that may never come. Trust me, I would love a good miracle. All I can say is the brain is not very resilient to injury or disease, especially as we age. The chances of a miracle are really, really small. I hate to be a Debby Downer, but the person could also be suffering as we are waiting for the miracle. No pressure of course, just one more factor to make you feel more guilty. Oh, and psychiatrists never charge for extra guilt. It's free.

Dementia and Denial

Issues with hospice are even more complicated for those with de- mentia. Let us explore that a moment. Dementia is a terminal ill- ness. There is no debate there. The debates generally arise when families disagree among themselves and with doctors if Grandma really has dementia. There can be a very lengthy period of denial of the illness before there is acceptance for both the resident and the family. Actually the statistic is that the diagnosis is often delayed until the middle stages of the disease. It is even more difficult when the denial continues into the later stages, which also is not uncom- mon. I totally understand this later denial as even I had it when my mother was obviously dying in front of my eyes.

I want us to do better for the declining person with demen- tia. I feel bad that they may be suffering as we are struggling with denial. They should not have to wait for us. We end up delaying comfort measures when they may be suffering. I can't force a family out of denial, but maybe we as medical professionals need to do a better job educating on dementia. And we need to understand the patient's wishes before they die. It will possibly prevent unneces- sary and ineffective care. For example, I have had families ask to withdraw pain meds to dementia patients so they can be more alert to do therapy. You know how hard it is for the physical therapist to push people who are suffering? Even the patients with dementia will beg us to stop doing the therapy. They will swing at us and curse us as well. We need to understand their illness to make the best decisions for them.

Breakdowns in Communications: A Big Mac for Gramps

Hesitant medical professionals are only part of the issue on starting hospice. Getting everyone on the same page is a big task. We have so much thrown on us as doctors, and these conversations sometimes take weeks. Sometimes, we also feel we are giving the answers, but they fall on deaf ears. It is easy as a doctor to become complacent or avoid conflict. Maybe the family is angry with our honesty and shuts us down. There are many ways in which the process fails. Once everyone finally is on the same page—that someone is suffering from dementia—then we all struggle when to start the comfort measures. As dementia is a terminal illness, a patient with dementia technically would qualify for hospice. But at what point do you determine that they are within that "six months to live" time frame? It is close to impossible to predict.

Sometimes hospice will tell you they can initiate services once a person starts failing to eat, also called "failure to thrive." Obviously, if a person stops eating, then their death is easier to predict. Most patients with dementia will eventually reach the stage when they lose the desire to eat. Should we do hospice then? Again, not a very simple answer. I notice that the thought of a loved one no longer wanting to eat is very scary for families. They fear the person is starving and suffering. In reality, they are not asking for food at all. They do not want to eat. They are annoyed we are even trying to get them to eat. I tell people that the minute Gramps asks for a Big Mac, I'll be on my way to McDonalds. Of course, in our food-based society, we panic and feel like we are going to kill the patient. Death by starvation. The tube in the stomach issue is the next discussion. I hold my breath and hope they do not start feeding through a tube. No one has ever shown feeding tubes to prolong or improve the quality of life. Any doctor will tell you that tubes should only be used in reversible medical illness. Dementia is not a reversible illness.

Of course sometimes as quickly as they stop eating, they rebound and fool everyone. This is where the struggle comes with hospice for dementia. The person has a bad week and "looks" like they are declining, goes on hospice for six months, improves and is taken off hospice. I can't tell you how many times I have heard,

"You just have to go on hospice temporarily. If they improve, they can come off hospice." For this reason, we have spent thousands of Medicare dollars in this dance. That would be great if there was actually some benefit to the patient. I just do not see it. If anything, it seems a bit like an expensive emotional roller coaster.

Dementia and Medicare

It does not seem like the best use of our Medicare resources. Apparently Medicare agrees as well: they are watching hospice to be sure they are not raking in the profits by starting hospice too early and for too long. I know, it sounds funny—people making a profit off death. Welcome to capitalism. We have a hospice in town whose top executive took home nearly six million in compensation. Really, is helping someone die that lucrative? Apparently so—you can Google it. Yes, there are some hospice programs that keep people with dementia, who are clearly not dying, on hospice too long. I have asked homes multiple times, "Why is James still on hospice?" Then there is silence afterward. It's an unspoken answer. You can probably guess by my phrasing, I do not feel hospice is the ideal option for dementia. Predicting death of a dementia resident is an art that is nearly impossible to master. We need to stop trying. I have tried and I personally stink at it. Oh yes, everyone else stinks at it too.

You may agree or disagree, but I feel the nursing homes should be able to deal with death and dementia without the hospice being involved. Follow my logic. We all know there is an obvious increase in your chance of dying if you have dementia. The average life span is seven years. Instead of trying to predict when the end is near, since we are obviously terrible at it, why can't we formulate a general game plan from the start? The conversations about death and dying need to come up as soon as the person moves into the home. It doesn't have to be the first conversations, but sometime in the first six months. It does not have to be with the person with the dementia, as many times they are not processing information well. Once the family and the facility are on the same page, we need to take it to the next level. The state surveyor, lawyers, Medicare/Medicaid auditors need to understand our plan. If they don't go along with it, it will fail. So what is the plan? They need to allow the home/family to choose a group of residents with dementia who will be allowed the freedom to decline. Oh yes, the freedom to say no more interventions. There will be no hospice roller coaster. No nursing home "tags" as someone had a bad outcome. No fears of a lawyer subpoena! We can finally be free to give the care we would like. We can help to stop suffering. You can say I am a dreamer, but I hope I am not the only one.

A Trip to the ER

For example, I had one family refuse to let their dad go to the hospital to evaluate shortness of breath. They were just sick of hospitals. They were tired of their dad getting more confused each time he went. It was understandable. Well, the home then became anxious that they would be sued if there were a bad outcome. What if he died as a result of not going to an emergency room? The family was interfering with care! They then told the family, either send him to the hospital, or put them him on hospice. Why? Because bad outcomes are expected in hospice. Hospice is just representing to everyone that it's ok to decline or die. The lawyers understand it; the state surveyors understand it as well. A decline basically sends nursing homes into panic. Homes feel a family can't have it both ways. So, it's on to hospice if you refuse the ER. As you can imagine, that goes down like a lead weight with a family. Not only are the families are upset their dad is sick, the next thing you know they need to be on hospice. They say, "I don't want hospice. Dad is not dying." They are correct technically. Dad is not dying, but he may if he does not go to the ER. I see both points of view, and there has to be a better plan. We have to create a possibility where it's fine to decline treatment without fear of repercussions. It would not be called "hospice." Maybe we can call it the "freedom to grow old without doctors bugging me plan? You can call it what you want, but not the word "hospice."

In order to get this plan to work, we can get all parties involved to agree there will be no aggressive interventions, constant blood draws, tubes, or hospitalization. We could even use medical marijuana and pain medications without fears of lawsuits over a fall or decline. We need the family, the home, the state, and the lawyers to all know our plan is to keep a person comfortable as they have their inevitable decline. It does not even matter how long the decline may take. So, for example, if a person does not want to eat and is loosing weight, we do not panic. We do not say to the family, you have to put in a feeding tube or we have to start hospice. You say, bring in their favorite foods and we will try to feed them. If not, we will just keep them happy with whatever they are willing to eat.

Fear of Discussing the Big "D"

Well, it is possibly an impossible goal. There are problems with my idea, I understand. We would all have to be comfortable with the subject of death. Few want to discuss death and dying, and I have lost track of the number of times families have asked me not to mention the word death out loud. It is as if I say the word, it may actually happen. It is also feared that even mentioning this word may cause people to give up on life. People are just as uncomfortable if I ask about suicide. One of my friends was accused of traumatizing a resident by just asking if they had any suicidal thoughts. Apparently she could have induced her to be suicidal by just asking the question. For my plan to work, we need to be able to discuss death as comfortably as asking people if they want ketchup or mustard on their hot dog. We all need to decide to stop freaking out at this word if we are really going to serve our elderly well. It's only uncomfortable if you make it that way. I have had some very intelligent and well thought out conversations with elderly about death. I hate to tell the many sons and daughters out there, but they are hiding their thoughts from you. They don't want to upset you. Most people after seventy know there is a possibility of dying, so it really should not be a scary terrible word to mention. Many times, I can only ask about death in secret because I really want to know how a person feels. I just say, "Have you had any thoughts about dying, any fears of dying?" I may be the only person who allows them to discuss their fears. We are all dying eventually—we need to stop fearing the conversation.

If you do not believe me, ask Buddha. That chubby little guy has great insights. Let me throw one at you: "It is better to spend one day contemplating the birth and death of all things than a hundred years never contemplating beginnings and endings." Let's not forget Henry Vandyke, that little smarty-pants. He says, "Some people are so afraid to die that they never begin to live." Death is really only a word; the meaning of death is something we attach. You can make it something to look forward to, like relief of suffering. It may also be a really cool place to visit, like a permanent vacation? Or something horrible like you will burn in hell fire. How do we know it's not some great awesome place, and we are afraid for no reason? Like I said, we need to think of the discussion of death as no scarier than a waitress asking if you want cream or sugar in your coffee.

You may disagree, but it's what I am personally shooting to attain. Look at the Dalai Lama—he is a smart a guy. Even he says, "There are only two things to do in life on the subject of death. Either you choose to ignore it—in which case you might be lucky enough to chase it away for a while—or you confront this prospect, you try to analyze it, and by doing so you try to diminish certain inevitable sufferings it causes." Of course, he does not believe you really die. Death to him was like leaving behind old clothing. He must think we are all a bit nutty in the West.

So, if we can conquer our fear of the subject, how would my new plan work? What kind of questions should we ask upon admission to a home? If someone has dementia, we need to ask what do to do if a person stops eating? Do we want to worry about their high cholesterol, take pills and draw labs to keep it under control? Or, do we let them eat pizza in peace? What do we do if they develop serious behavioral issues? Would you do what it takes to keep them out of a psychiatric hospital? Do we try to resuscitate them each time their heart stops? Are we going to replace a heart valve for the patient to live longer, but potentially to advance their dementia? The questions are endless really. We may have to decide as we go, but always trying to decide what makes a person happy. I had one dementia unit where every patient had significant obvious dementia. Almost each of those patients was full code. This means that we were going to keep them alive at all costs. If their heart stopped, we were going to pump the chest, shock the heart, intubate their lungs, and keep them alive. Yes, even if you had no idea what was going on, we wanted you around. You need to live a little longer in our home. Let that thought sink in for a moment. Pretty much 99 percent of patients will say they do not want to live in a home, and we are going to extend your stay. That's like a hotel from hell with no checkout desk. My favorite home, called Golden Beers Nursing and Rehab, had almost every resident with significant dementia a "do not resuscitate." This was because the head nurse, named Jean, had those hard conversations with all families. She had a rough smoker's voice and spiky hair. She even confided to me once she liked sex clubs as a younger woman. I loved that. She had many wrinkles reflecting her years of experience as well as the number of cigarettes she smoked. She told families she was not going to be resuscitating someone with a terminal illness in so many words. I never heard a family complain about her request. She was good. She was smooth, like butter.

Despite how good an idea my plan seems to me (to continually prepare for the end) there is one more way in which it may fail.

Doctors and nurses are too hesitant to have these conversations. It's hard to find more Jeans since she retired. Many avoid these conversations like the plague. To entice us back, Medicare has recently announced it will pay us to have "end of life" discussions with people. This is a new development. This seems interesting at first, unless you want to be called a "death panel." Yes, I watch the news and know what the Republicans are saying. I know where you are trying to push all us doctors—on death panels, dammit. We will be accused of trying to ration out health care to those who have the best chance to survive. We are going to throw grandma off a cliff! I appreciate the government wanting us to get more involved, but hey, toss us a bone. Can you at least give us some lawsuit relief? Without this, I fear few doctors will take up the Medicare push to have us discuss end of life issues. I suppose if you offered a lot of money to have the discussion, doctors would be helping you write your bucket lists. I am thinking the current offer is not going to change the situation greatly. In the meantime, we probably will have those discussions with families who want to have the conversation. For those families who are too anxious to discuss, the conversation will be about as uncomfortable as having a hemorrhoid lasered. Not that I know anything about this particular procedure personally. I am just saying it's easier for us to discuss flowers, bunnies, and babies than death.

The Profiteers

There is one more issue that I need to mention. I only mention it as it could also throw a wrench in my plan. It is about money and greed and the way in which it drives the system to do more care. Not from hospice, but from the nursing homes themselves. Follow my train of thought: the advances in medical care have made the actual care a very expensive endeavor. The drug companies profit from our chronic illnesses. The number of elderly is going to skyrocket as the baby boomers hit old age. We spend a tremendous amount of money on the last few months of life, more than any other times in life. Medicare is not going to be able to continue to pay for all these costs—it will go bankrupt. We, as a society, expect and demand the highest levels of care. This all is a set up for eventual disaster. I am pretty sure we are going to blow the whole Medicare money wad soon. We can only go on this path for so long, before we have nothing left.

So where does the greed come in? There is this thing called "skilled" Medicare benefits. Let me explain. Say your mom is admitted to a hospital for an acute medical event. She will be entitled to get "skilled" Medicare benefits if she stays in the hospital for three midnights. Once she is "skilled," she can then go live in a nursing home and get physical therapy, occupational therapy, and a bunch of other therapies. Therapy to strengthen her for her return home. "Skilled" residents pay the nursing home a nice chunk of change, a major part of their profits. The consumer also benefits from the twenty-four hour nursing and monitoring. It sounds great if you are just in a home short term. But what about for those residents who live in nursing homes long term who end up in the hospital? Homes take advantage of this three-midnight renewal of skilled benefits in the following way: The long term resident with dementia develops pneumonia. They spend at least three days in the hospital and come back skilled. The home now can use up more skilled benefits. Can you say "cha ching?" They are still trying to rehabilitate declining confused residents. They will use as much of the benefit as possible, and try to document the necessity for Medicare. Trust me, I have spoken to many therapists who are trying to perform the therapy. Many are disgusted over the waste of Medicare money. They do not always have a say in when enough is enough. If they want to keep the job, they do the work. Some are so turned off, they leave the home. I just asked a therapist yesterday, "who pressures you more to do therapy that seems to lack benefit, families or the nursing home? She looked all anxious as if I was some auditor trying to get someone in trouble. She knew exactly what I was talking about. I had to rephrase the question, "Ok, every home but his home we are in right now." Her sphincter noticeable relaxed and she responded, "Both do equally." I would have guessed more the homes personally. However, the nursing homes are doing it for profit, and families do it, as they love their parents. I told you I would be honest, I know it sounds bad but it's true. Greed is prolonging care.

What is even more confusing to me are those residents who go from skilled therapy benefits, and then placed directly into hospice. We did all this work to improve them; then we let them die? It makes no sense. If you think they belong on hospice from the beginning, why are you torturing them with physical therapy? Therapy is really hard when you are eighty- or ninety-years old. It's even harder if you are confused. The residents can't complain about all the therapy, as they are "incompetent dementia residents." They do not always have a voice. I think the answer to the therapy to hospice issue is obvious: greed from homes and no one wanting to mention hospice until homes have done a ton of therapy. The fact of the matter is, therapy does not cure serious illness, but we spend money on it like it does. Well, Medicare is aware and is trying to crack down. Of course, there should be whistle blower protection if a therapist wants to make a living. In the meantime, the excessive therapy just gives false hope to families and may again prolong suffering. Even if a dementia resident does have some benefit from the therapy, it quickly disappears after they stop doing the therapy. Many may agree or disagree. I can only share my personal experiences. I have this one resident named Ann. Every time she sees me, she asks when therapy is going to make her walk. She is so confused. We all know she will never get the therapy. Even if she did, she would never be able to walk. What I do know is that if Ann spends three nights in the hospital, she will be back on therapy regardless.

Drug Companies and Skippy Peanut Butter

I know it is not a huge revelation that there is greed in nursing homes. I have even seen homes threaten to stop giving doctors new patients if they try to cancel skilled benefits too quickly and opt for hospice. You will never survive as a doctor in a home if you deem a resident incapable of benefitting from physical therapy before a home is ready to give up the skilled Medicare money. Oh yes, let's not leave out the drug companies. I just personally witnessed a name brand drug representative come to one of my dementia units. She wanted to review all the patients' charts to see who would qualify to start on Namenda. If I have not mentioned it before, Namenda is the medication that really seems to do little for end-stage dementia in my experience. The drug company says it may slow down a decline in cognition. I say "long shot." I kept my mouth shut as the rep babbled on, which if you know me is not an easy task. The Namenda drug rep let us know she was given permission by the medical director of the nursing home to find customers. "Can I just look through these charts to see who may benefit from the medications? Really? I am pretty sure that looks on the outside like a drug company preying on confused elderly. I was proud of my nurse who refused to allow her in the charts. We can't make decisions based on who will become rich. We can't make decisions as doctors based on who will like us more. Who will buy us better drug lunches? We need to make decisions based on what is best for our patients. I recall being in a drug review meeting in one of my homes. It is a meeting where we try to reduce the psychiatric medications of all the residents. There was an infamous pharmacist present who is known for getting the drug representative to provide a free meal to meeting. At one point, I was pressured by this pharmacist to start using their drug more often in the home "unless you want peanut butter and jelly sandwiches for lunch." I happen to really like peanut butter and jelly, so I got up and walked out on his un-ethical, slimy meeting. Go Skippy Peanut Butter! I then called the pharmacy, where he worked, and let them know my mother made us peanut butter and jelly sandwiches all the time. No one says bad things about peanut butter and jelly or tells me what drugs to prescribe mister. Let's keep the drug companies out of the homes.

The homes contribute to the problem in other ways. So many times I wanted to be honest with families. Nursing homes do not always allow for this honesty. Nursing homes are a business when it comes down to it. We don't want to piss off the customers. We want to make them happy, even if the ideas the families come up with seem impossible. We are forever ordering tests and scans as if somehow they are actual cures for an illness. Each person deserves one brain scan. However, repeated scans are hard to perform on confused people and rarely offer a change in care. All tests should be done only with the thought of (1) will it will improve quality of life, or (2) decrease the suffering of a patient. They should not be done to make happy customers or to avoid lawsuits. I have been told, just "order it so they will leave us alone." We have to resist that urge. We need to tell people a test is not going to help change care or benefit a resident.

Empathy

Well, I think I have ranted on for some time now. I wanted to give the multiple reasons why I feel we have trouble just keeping people comfortable. We are all to blame in one way, shape, or form. We need to all introspect on our own. I would love a place for people to go to just have the freedom to do what they want as they decline. It is for selfish reasons as well. What if I get dementia? I do not want to live in homes the way they are now. I would love to have a place, that if I became demented, I could go out with a bang. There is no shame at throwing in the towel when your body has had enough. All you are saying is you are tired of suffering. If you are tired of watching your loved one suffer, it's fine to let them go as well.

One last thought as we leave this chapter. I started the chapter by asking why we still have trouble letting go. I leave you with a little test for those who are struggling with the guilt and fear of letting their loved one go. Besides the QQ equation, I have used one other simple test to decide when enough is enough. It is a personal test only you can answer. This test has to be done in a relaxed state. Without another thought, you have to respond to a specific question I will ask you now. If you even add your own rational mind, the test is invalid. If you start to judge your feelings, it also invalidates the test. The test is one simple question. Ask yourself, if you were actually in your loved ones shoes, would you want to live the life they have now? Your first response is the most intuitive and honest I feel. You may not like the first answer you pick, but it is usually correct. You have to be willing to follow your gut feeling. You can try this first response test if you are ever in a position to have to make a medical decision for a loved one and are struggling with the "right" answer. If you are unable to imagine being in their shoes, you have to consider the thought of letting go—letting go not as a failure or weakness but as an act of love.

Let me give you a real life example. I had a ninety-year-old woman named Rita I treated a year ago. She was living independently until the frequent falls started. She was just placed in the one of the homes where I came to meet her. From the moment she arrived at the home, she did poorly. She was declining quickly from dehydration and a bladder infection. She was no longer able to converse. I spent time with her daughter, who was given the option of intravenous fluids and antibiotics or letting her pass. If she chose the hospital for fluids, she would be poked and prodded again. If not, she would allow her mother to continue to slip deeper into a coma and die with hospice. What made her decision more complicated was that Rita had told her daughter she would rather die than live in a nursing home the rest of her days. If her daughter "cured" her infection and dehydration, her fate would be to live in a nursing home. Rita had already given her daughter the permission to let her go with her wishes. The daughter did not want to follow those wishes and pushed for the IV's. She could not imagine life without her mother. Well, Rita died before we could intervene. She did have her wish met. She did not have to spend the rest of her days in a nursing home. Sometimes, our own wants and desires cloud our judgment for those we love.

I often wondered how people died hundreds of years ago. Well, they died: it was ok. They did not have all our hundreds of options. It is so complicated now. I am trying to uncomplicate the situation. You may have disagreed with me on many points, but I at least maybe made you think from a different perspective.

CHAPTER 8

Letting Go, Part 2

➤ Analysis for psychiatrists.
➤ The problem of the "gifted child."
➤ Narcissism.
➤ Learning from one's own family.
➤ Seeking approval from one's parents.
➤ Learning to say "no."
➤ Resolving emotional issues from childhood.

Being a psychiatrist, I have to analyze everything. It's what we do. I don't analyze the stuff most people would probably think. I'm too tired to figure out everyone's personality. I also do not read minds like people imagine. And yes, they do imagine. So what do I analyze? Well, in the previous chapter, I looked at the external reasons why people have difficulty letting go. Now I will do what shrinks love to do, look at the internal reasons that make it hard to let go. In other words, I want to shrink you, my reader. Well, I can at least make you think about your situation in different ways. Therapy is like making the perfect al dente spaghetti. You just keep throwing pieces to the wall and see what sticks. Well, this is what I am going to do—throw out some ideas. If you like the idea, throw a little cheese on it, and eat it up. If it tastes a little tough, feel free to throw it back in the pot.

The Shrink Gets Shrunk: Me! A Narcissist?

I feel the best way to explain my point is to start by sharing more of my personal journey. I mentioned my mother in the beginning of the book for good reason. Now I have to finish our story. After her death, I completed medical school and went on to psychiatry residency. In our training, we were pushed to have our own therapy. It helped us learn to separate our own issues from the issues of our patients. My counselor was a cool Rhode Island guy, but a little eccentric at the same time. Shocking that a psychiatrist is eccentric, huh? He had cash, and he decorated his home office well. Even his cats looked cool—and very well adjusted. They probably had had therapy too. After a few meetings, he let me know I had some degree of narcissism and that I needed to read a certain book. It was only after my second session. He basically called me an asshole and sent me out to read a book? Nice! Therapy was not what I imagined it would be. One of the worst things to be called in psychiatry is narcissistic. It was a blow to my gigantic ego. I finally fell off my high horse. Okay, I'm being sarcastic; I didn't see it. I really thought hard about it and researched all the definitions of narcissism. What is this guy talking about? All I could come up with is maybe I could be a wee bit over critical of others and also had trouble taking criticism? I would think most people would be narcissistic then if you define it this way. So I am normal narcissistic? Well, at least he was not quite referring to the type of narcissism I was used to hearing about, the type like Donald Trump. He is so stuck on himself that he will crucify anyone who critiques him. Yeh, I am not that bad, although I do wish I had a personal lawyer who would sue anyone who pisses me off. As you can see, my mind was spinning.

Ann Miller's Theories

So, I read the book he told me to get and played along with his little game. Plus, he came strongly recommended by one of my professors, so I couldn't blow him off. The book was called, *Drama of the Gifted Child* by Ann Miller (1981). The book was very short when I picked it up. I was pretty happy it was small, as I did not like to read. The book, however, was so dry and boring, I had to almost tie myself to a chair to read it. I chugged slowly through it and absorbed the ideas. Who am I kidding? My attention span was not able to handle reading the whole tortuous thing. I did learn a great deal from what I did finish. I found the book could explain my whole mother-daughter relationship in a way that finally made sense to me. It was my life in a nutshell. Apparently, I was a gifted child according to my therapist. I liked that. I knew I was gifted somehow. Okay, well, he explained it more, and I wasn't gifted in the way I'd imagined. Damn him, couldn't he throw me one bone already? Gifted children are gifted in that they can figure out everything their mothers' need and want to be happy. I suppose you can call it being intuitive or empathic. Gifted children are experts at watching and listening to see what makes their parents' happy. It is not at a conscious level, but there are always messages parents send to children about what emotions or feelings are more or less acceptable. Let me quote Ann Miller, who, of course, is way more serious and not half as funny as I am.

"The child that is hidden behind her achievements wakes up and asks: What would happen if I had appeared before you sad, needy, angry, furious? Where would your love have been then? And I was all these things as well. Does this mean it was not really me who you loved, but only what I pretended to be? The well-behaved, reliable, empathetic, understanding and convenient child, who was in fact never a child at all? From the beginning I have been a little adult. My abilities were then simply misused."

I know, this woman is serious. Glad she was not my therapist. I like her ideas, but she sounds as if she needs a martini and a relaxing foot rub. She is basically saying kids have a natural empathy that makes them gifted, and some parents rely on it. In the end, the children will hide unacceptable parts of themselves to get their parents' love. As a result, they are never able to find their true selves. This can result in feelings of emptiness and depression later in life.

Narcissus

Well then what does this all have to do with being narcissistic? It does not seem narcissistic of me to want to please my parents. It is, however, narcissistic to rely on others to help maintain your self-image. Let's dig a bit deeper into Ann Miller's ideas—the narcissism topic in particular. You may have heard about Narcissus, a mythological Greek youth who became infatuated with his own reflection in a lake. He did not realize at first that it was his own reflection, but when he did, he died. Apparently, he wanted that imaginary person to love him so badly that he could not take it any longer when they disappeared. Yes, he was in love with his puddle reflection. Kind of a sad story. I guess the sun came out and dried up all the rain that day. A bad day for Narcissus. It was his whole identity—that little puddle. So, his self worth was based on something outside of himself. That was a bad spot to be in: don't be that guy. We have to rely on ourselves for our self-image; this can never evaporate.

So in Ann Miller's theory, the narcissist is the parent, and the puddle is their child. Follow me; I swear it's more logical than Freud's theories on anal fixations. So why do people decide to have children in the first place? There are many healthy reasons obviously to have children, but I only want you to focus on one not so healthy reason: when someone with decreased self image wants to have a child. Could they possibly be trying to create that little puddle buddy? Think about it. What if you had low self-esteem? Most narcissistic people do have low self-image to different degrees. How can you repair that self image unconsciously? Wouldn't it be nice to have a child who loved you? They would think you are the bee's knees, give you total attention. This kid could be as smart as you, as good looking, and maybe even better in sports than you. Everyone will admire your kids and say what a great pool of genes you possess. Yeah baby, look what I made! The baby can't run away from you; they are totally dependent on you for everything. Your puddle can't just up and disappear; it's your child. Your boss, your mom, your spouse can all reject you and leave you. Children have to stay and thrive. They may run from you later in life when they are able, but they are with you in the beginning. Children crave a parent's love and acceptance so they want to please. It's a perfect set up really. The question is, what are children willing to give up to get that approval. Will they learn to hide thoughts, feelings, and emotions a parent finds unacceptable. Does the gifted child lose her true self in the process of becoming the ideal child? She may lock away her true feelings. Later in life, her self worth will be based on people outside herself.

This is the narcissism my therapist was talking about with me. My mother trained me to support her self-image, and in return I was relying on others to support my self-image. When she thought I was wonderful, my world was great. When she was sad, I was anxious. I felt responsible. I knew when I was very young that my mother was depressed, and I tried so hard to take her pain from her. She didn't come to me asking me to help her obviously, but my "gift" was my empathy and sensitivity. Ann Miller says it better: "Many people suffer all their lives from this oppressive feeling of guilt, the sense of not having lived up to their parents expectations. This feeling is stronger than any intellectual insight they may have, that it is not a child's task or duty to satisfy a parent's needs. No argument can overcome these guilt feelings, for they have their beginnings in life's earliest periods, and from that they derive their intensity."

Again, obviously all this occurs at more at unconscious levels. My mother didn't say, "Come here and help me with my problems," although I have met mothers who have done that to their kids. Also, I really do not feel Ann Miller is trying to lay a guilt trip on all parents and accuse them of using their children. I feel she is really trying to break an unhealthy cycle. I also do not think most people would notice these patterns unless they really thought about it; I know I never did before writing this book. Now I am always thinking about them, especially when I interact with my own children. I find it actually very useful. I weigh a lot of my decisions based on, "Am I making this choice as I want my children to love me and not be angry with me, or am I making it as I know it is what is best for them?" I ask if all my readers would consider really looking to see if these patterns exist for them with their parents, even at a minor level. If they do, I promise they will come up frequently as you have to make end-of-life decisions for another family member. It may even come up between husbands and wives as well. My therapist always did say you marry someone similar to your parents in some way. I know, creepy.

Examples from My Family: Big Brother Jim

Since this can be a confusing concept, let me give you some examples of the drama. Then I think it will be clear why I feel these issues arise in making end-of-life decisions. I mentioned my older brother Jim who always felt as if he failed my mother. He wanted to be a journalist when he was young. He told me my mother frowned upon the profession. Not only did she feel it was not a worthy profession, but she compared him to my brother Ray. Why couldn't he be like Ray, the physicist—that is a real career.What choice did he have? He wanted my mother to love him. Jim had to close down that part of himself who wanted to write and hide it in order to get the love he wanted from my mother. He never pursued journalism. I recall him always talking about going to law school instead. I knew when I was quite young that my brother was always sad. I never knew why until this year. You see, he had disappeared from our family for twenty years. We all presumed him dead, and I guess in a way, part of him had died. When he resurfaced, he told me the story of such severe rejection that he had hidden from all of us. He could not handle one more negative comment. I am finally getting to know my real brother. He sent me what he has been writing. He is the journalist now that he was once told was not acceptable. He blossomed in an environment where no one let him know that what he wanted was not good enough. He found his authentic self. In the process, he had also fought off stage four throat cancer, so I am lucky cancer did not take away my opportunity to know him. He reconnected with me as I was just finishing this book, and I am so incredibly happy I can tell the world how really proud I am of him.

I also found it interesting to see how my mother had impacted my whole family so differently. My sister struggled with self-image issues as well, but she was so much more protective of my mother. My mother was so poor at hearing criticism as to her it meant rejection and also that we did not love her. I noticed that my sister was never comfortable pointing out my mother's weaknesses. I always wanted to tell her our mother was not perfect, no one is perfect! I thought maybe we could bond over the issue. My mother trained her well. If my mother's self image were better, she could handle the criticism we had of her parenting style. My brother Ray seemed the same as my sister. He would protect her to a fault and even physically. Once Ray was so angry I had upset my mother, he chased me out of the house. Really? What daughter has not upset their mother as a teenager, pretty normal. You would think I was smoking pot and blowing it in my mother's face the way he acted. I guess she trained him to be a great bodyguard. I know I am not imagining this, as my mother would try to get me in the same spot. She would scream my name when the fights between my father and her went out of control. I was a tomboy and bad ass as well, so I assume that's why I was called for the physical stuff. Regardless, we were the protectors of her self-esteem and at times her safety. The reason I find this interesting is I have many clients that refuse to say anything negative about their parents. If I probe a little, you can see the protective anger come out and the subject is closed. I always have a little internal questions of whether they also were trained to protect their parents' self image. It is impossible not to have a fault dammit. We can't deal without dramas until we all agree on this fact.

The Softball Team

Let me give a few more examples. I really want my readers to understand the concepts. I will again use my own personal examples of the drama. In exchange, I expect you all to be just as vulnerable. The truth shall set you free! I recall playing for the girl's softball team in middle school. All the players would wear corduroy pants and team shirts on our game days. We wanted to stand out to the other students as cool. I wanted so badly to wear those stupid corduroy pants. They came in all these awesome colors and they matched different shirts. Finally, she agreed to let me wear the pants! Oh yeah, I had the outfit ready to go! The day finally came for me to put them on and I couldn't do it. I was so upset with the thought of disappointing her. We were religious, and pants were, I suppose, a bit heathen. If I wore those pants, I thought she would not love me the same. So, I forced myself to wear the same boring skirts and face the rejection at school. I am sure it was one of those horrible wrap round skirts too. There was no way I was going to risk having her disappointed in me, so I wrapped it on me. I quit the team shortly thereafter. I felt really sad that day.

A Deep Secret

I had actually hid a much deeper secret from my mother, a very big part of my identity. It turns out, I was having major crushes on girls as young as third grade. I was in love with Mrs. Munson. In love at that age just meant it felt good to look at her. I even recall having this little girl named April come up to me in third grade to complain I was staring at her too much. Damn, that stunk. She was so cute. I never looked in her general direction again. I was so embarrassed. Regardless, I had all these emotions and feelings I hid out of shame and fear of rejection. I was terrified for years someone would discover my horrible secret. I tried hard to date boys to make my family not worry about me. God, I felt I could kiss a cereal box and have more pleasure than kissing a boy. I just never wanted my mother to feel she failed by having a gay daughter. In case you are wondering, she died not knowing that secret. I did not want my truth to kill her.

Unfortunately, this constant desire to make her happy planted something else in me. It planted the seeds of anger toward her, an anger that she would not love me for who I was inside. As I grew older, I no longer wanted to be around her. Later, when she developed cancer, the anger turned into isolation from her. An anger that kept me emotionally distant from her when we needed each other the most. She was again trying to rely on me emotionally as she was dying, and I was done feeling used. I just watched at a distance as she withered away. I just wanted her suffering to be over, and for her to die. It felt horrible to say that as I loved her, but I wanted her pain to end.

Later, I often wondered if her tremendous fight to live was more related to a fear of death and a fear of leaving her children alone. Would her many life-prolonging procedures been cancelled if she felt more comfortable with dying. We never were close enough to have those talks. All I am sure of is that I felt completely separate from her, as she died, each of us on our own little island. I had to resolve my anger at her well after she died. It was eventually replaced with empathy for what she had to suffer in her childhood, as well as what I had to suffer in mine.

Pleasing Parents

I would see many of the same situations in my nursing homes, with both sons and daughters doing what I would do as a daughter. Children trying to do the impossible to please parents. For example, children who didn't want to let their parents down by even placing them in a nursing home in the first place. Of course, they had no choice but to place them for various reasons. They would tell me with long guilty faces, "I promised her I would never do that." I have had children tell me threats they received from parents, "If you place me, then you are the worst child ever and I will disown you." They will just make you feel horribly guilty. Listen to me now. You all need to stop making this promise. It may be impossible for you to keep it! I don't care how strong you are; even the strongest will wilt in the face of watching your confused parent twenty-four hours a day/ seven days a week. If you can do it or arrange for someone else to do it, then skip this section. If you are forced to have to place you parents in a home for health or economic reasons, stop feeling like a total failure and place them. For the kid wrapped up in the drama (my word for the concept of the book), the rejection is too much to bear and you will promise your parents all kinds of things you can't produce. I know you do not want to let them down, you may feel like that kid again who failed. You will neglect your own health and family to unhealthy degrees. You will hear everyone and their mother tell you to "take time for yourself." Of course, that will annoy you each time you hear it. Do not let your fear of letting your parents down, drive your life into the ground. Next time, just say I will do my best to keep you at home and out of a nursing home. This is more realistic and authentic answer. It is the truth. Parents deep down inside have to know this somewhere.

I am a mother of three children. It's going to be a cold day in hell if you think I will ask my children to take care of me when I am old. I believe, since I turned eighteen, that I became responsible for myself forever and ever. I refuse to burden my kids. If they want to be burdened, then cool, that is different. I'm staying on your couch. I get the remote. But, I personally need to plan for the possibility I will end up in a nursing home all by myself. I will have to put my big girl Depends on and deal with it. Will I be hurt if they do not let me move in? Well, of course it will hurt a little. However, I will not have my kids lose a job, or develop health issues, to avoid placing me in a home. This is just my humble opinion. You may think that sounds harsh, especially for those who feel children should take care of their parents in old age. You know what? Let me add a side note to make you feel better. Something I have noticed is the elderly who have always tried to love their children unconditionally, get the most attention later on. Parents who used guilt to get their children to conform, seem to get the least help later on. The help needs to come naturally, not forced. Children want to help when they are not pressured or guilted. It's a bit of reverse psychology.

The drama issues are much more complicated if you are dealing with a loved one with dementia. Another reason why we need to do this work early in the illness. I have explained how people with dementia lose their reasoning and logical abilities. Well, all these discussions should happen before they lose their logic. Otherwise, if you try placing them in a home, best prepare for some real rejection. They will yell at you, accuse you of stealing their money, and hate you forever. They will make you feel like beans on toast; you will taste bad, look bad, and smell bad. They will never recall when you visit them and accuse you of never coming. They are mentally not able to understand your desire to keep them safe and happy as they decline. Be prepared to be hated. Because if you are still relying on your parents for your self-image, you will not make the best decisions for them. Slowly removing someone's independence is going to be a horrible process no matter what you do to prepare. But, maybe not quite so bad if you can separate yourself out from the drama. You have to prepare to face constant rejection from your parents.

The Perils of Denial

If you think about all this, I can totally get why people want to deny their parent has dementia. If you finally accept what is going on, you have to face these situations. It sounds God-awful. However, if you continue to avoid the situation, you may risk putting your loved one in a potentially dangerous situation. You will leave them alone in their homes longer than is safe, as you do not want to upset them. The next thing you know, a cop is calling saying they found your mother wandering in a 7-Eleven. No amount of Slurpee can brighten that situation. You may also let them take their own medications at their insistence, until they have an accidental over-dose. All these decisions will be ultimately be yours, but you need to be aware of all the emotional factors impacting them. More examples, "I can't take the car keys from Dad; he will hate me." So the alternative is he accidentally harms himself or others on the road? You may have to be the bad guy and take the spark plugs from his car. He will hate you, as he is not able to process why you are doing it. The same situation arises when you have to take the checkbook, or get them to see the doctor—the examples are endless. Get used to being hated. I have been called everything in the book. Now I just start accepting if people are not mad with me, then I am probably not helping them. Not too easy from a woman who needed a puddle buddy to feel good about themselves.

The drama can come up in daily health care decisions as I have said, but how does it come up in the dying process? As parents use their children as mirrors for their self-image, children can also be dependent on parents to make them feel secure as well. As a result, they may hold on to the dying parent at all costs. The family's struggles with letting go so much that they will then want the doctors to give more antidepressants, more medical tests, more therapy—just more. They just don't want to lose their parents. It is completely understandable. Just be cautious that the fear of losing someone is not driving your decisions. For example, I have had nursing home residents in their 80s and 90s beg the family to let them go. I know as they tell the family while I am standing there with them in the room. Yes, pretty awkward. But then, the family will say to me, "She doesn't know what she is saying." They try to shut down the conversation. Well, what if she says it a lot and not a little? I think then it might mean something? Sadly, I stink at pretending I did not hear something. I so wish I could do that sometimes. I prefer to discuss the elephant in the room, as it is too big to hide. I don't think anyone died because they were talking about dying. I suppose anything is possible, but unlikely. Ask yourself if you are telling them not to talk about dying because you are not able to cope with them leaving? If the answer is that you fear them dying more than helping them let go, then slow down and think about things again.

Unresolved Emotional Issues

I think you can possibly see how our unresolved emotional issues with our loved ones can cause us to prolong life unnecessarily. But, there is one more point Ann Miller makes about why we are not able to resolve these issues earlier. I think most would agree with her. We have, as a nation, cut ourselves off from our own feelings. Ann says, "People have all developed the art of not experiencing feelings, for only a child can experience her feelings only when there is somebody there who accepts her fully, understands her, and supports her. If that person is missing, if the child must risk losing the mother's love in order to feel, then she will repress her emotions. She cannot even experience them secretly, 'just for herself'; she will fail to experience them at all. But they will nevertheless stay in her body, in her cells, stored up as information that can be triggered by a later event."

Miller felt strongly that we have to get in touch with the emotions and feelings we have always hidden. We have become a nation of people afraid of experiencing our own feelings. As parents, our job is to help our children learn how to feel and express emotions. Not just feel them, express them. And when we express them, we should not be made to feel guilty or ashamed of having the feeling. I am not just talking about happy feelings—those are easy. I am discussing the hard feelings of anger, fear, sadness and insecurity. Just let kids say the feeling, empathize with it, and move on. We are not there to agree or disagree with their feelings, even if they make us uncomfortable. It's fine for them to feel disappointed when you say no, so let them feel it. If they are sad, don't give them a piece of candy to stop crying, listen to them and just be there. They want you, not chocolate. Let them feel without repercussions. They are not "babies," or "weak" if they have certain feelings; they are just little humans trying to figure it all out. If again, you know all this already and you had warm supportive parents, skip the chapter. Many have not had these positive experiences with their parents. Many are thrust into end-of-life decisions without the inner emotional compass.

I have noticed these emotional shut downs even more lately as I have been working more in the drug and alcohol field. Nowhere has the suppression of feelings been more obvious to me then there. Heroin is like brain Novocaine. I am thinking that many children are not taught how to regulate their emotions, so they use drugs to suppress, regulate, and numb. After they are finally detoxed, they are inundated with all kinds of feelings they are unable to manage. Obviously, there are other causes of addiction, but I place this up there with the most common. We stink as a culture at feeling our emotions. We get a strong anxiety, anger, or fear, and we are hitting the bottle, cigarettes, the sexual encounter, or the scratch ticket. Oh, and one I tried for a while, Super Mario. (I still love you Mario, even though we have not played together in a while.) We need to make time to learn to feel. I do not care the way in which it is done, as long as it is done.

I prefer therapy at least once, but you have to find the right therapist. You have to find the therapist who will challenge you to feel. You need to find one like I had—he pushed me. If therapy is not a work out of emotions, you are doing it wrong. You should be mentally exhausted by the end of the session. I had it rough. For example, I stunk so bad at expressing anger that my therapist would try to piss me off to get it out. It's a bit unorthodox actually, but he was working for my best interest. He was trying to teach me I could be angry with someone and still have them care about me. So powerful to have the experience and not just talk about it. I did not get what he was doing at first, so I just thought he was an ass. He would start our sessions by answering mail. A normal person would have told him to cut that out—this is time I paid for your attention. I could not express to this man that he was making me angry. I think I could do it now, but not at the time.

Using Your Own Experience to Help Others

I decided after all my soul searching and therapy, I was on a mission to help people feel emotions. Initially, I stunk at it. I was like a bull in a china shop. The emotion stuffers hated me. I was just trying to push them to feel, I guess I didn't explain what I was doing so well. Maybe it was my blunt style as well. I can't escape the Severson tell-it-like-it-is talk. I just felt so strongly that we have to know our emotions, as they are our internal compasses in life. I was really trying to help. I knew for me, my emotions were my compass in many ways. Healthy emotions and add in a little smidgen of intuition and common sense and the equation was complete. I can't imagine life without fully functioning feelings.

In addition to learning my own emotions as a doctor, I also had to learn to handle what intense emotions I brought out in others. I had one particular patient who was a lawyer and so deeply stoic. He dealt with his dying as a giant checklist. Every time anyone would speak to him, he would review his chart of symptoms, treatments, and care. I hated to see him coming, as he was so dry and boring. On the other hand, I felt so guilty not to listen to his spreadsheets, as I knew he was dying. Even his family was not able to emotionally connect with him. So I felt pressured to get him to feel his emotions before it was too late. I just told it straight, "I want to get to know how you feel; I can't relate to this other stuff. Stop talking about facts, I can't connect with that." Well, I did finally get an emotion. It was anger. I had something to work with finally, and then he fired me dammit. I had all these fantasies he would have this deep conversations with his sisters after our talk. Talk about a fantasy. I was not "meeting him where he was at" as my other teachers would tell me. About a month before he died, he asked to see me again. I never went to find out what he wanted. I feel bad to this day that I avoided finding him. I will never forget him as he helped me learn a big lesson. He reminded me again, I have to be able to handle the anger and the disappointment patients may show toward me for pushing them to feel. I had imagined he was going to tell me I was a terrible doctor for not wanting to see his lists. I was not warm and compassionate enough. I actually have no idea what he wanted to tell me; I made it up in my head. My drama was interfering with the care. I am hoping to this day, he understood I really cared about him by pushing him. So I am hoping that my readers can learn from my mistakes! Seize opportunities before they disappear in death.

I see another general trend lately that makes me even more nervous. There are not only some parents who are shaping children to reinforce their self-image but there are also parents who need their children's love so badly, they do not want to disappoint their children in any way. It's like a reverse Ann Miller. I see parents now too afraid to upset their children. If the child cries and screams over not having the toy they want, the parent gives in gives them what they want. Parents basically stink at saying no. I have been totally guilty of that with my toddler, so I am not trying to judge. For example, you know that screaming noise kids make when they do not get their way? It is one of the worst sounds God ever created, and I just need it to stop. I also just wanted the little crumb snatcher to be happy. My hardest time is at night, when I have to put her asleep alone in her bed. She cries and has that little orphan face. If I did not know any better, I would think she was dying. It sadly took me awhile to know she was playing me. She relaxes that look of angst for a split second and smiles. She is good. I assume it will be a lot worse as a teen. Parents are becoming too afraid to say no to their children. We let our children stay up to late, with electronics, of course. We complain to the doctor the children are tired, moody, and may have attention deficit disorder. All because we can't say, "Shut off the electronics and go to bed. Children have to have limits as it actually shows them you do care. I really think parents are this way as they fear rejection from the kids, or we will hurt their feelings. Allowing children to express feelings doesn't mean we let them manipulate bad ideas out of us. We have to be on our toes. Setting limits with them also teaches gratitude, something we risk losing in such a privileged nation

When Is Enough Enough?

What does this have to do with death and dying? Maybe I am getting paranoid, but I think every now and then, that the grown kid who can't hear the word "no" ends up making an end-of-life decision in one of my nursing home. I know the nurses will appreciate this point, and I may piss off a few customers with this next thought. If it was a rare occurrence, I would not even bother mentioning it here, but it is not rare. Let me share a common conversation I overhear. The conversation goes like this, between a physical thera-pist and a family member: "I want my mother to get more physical therapy." Therapist: "Well she has reached her maximum potential so she no longer will benefit. Once they max out, Medicare will not pay for it any longer." Family: "So you just don't want to pay for it? You can't stop it just because Medicare is not paying. She still needs the therapy." If you look in this example, you will see the person is unable to hear that "no" word in the correct way. They are so focused on the word "no" therapy, they miss the most important point the therapist is trying to make. The therapists are saying that they could do therapy on Mom until the cows came home and she still would not walk any better. The "no" is really coming from Mom's body, not Medicare and not the therapist.

The focus is, "I want what I want," and I will not take "no" for an answer, no matter how unreasonable. The medical field has become like a giant buffet table; people think they can just load up their plates. Doctors have become like the parents who can't say no, and they agree to the most outrageous requests to avoid the blow back. In order to succeed as a culture, and not waste all our precious resources, we have to hear the "no" word and accept it. Medicare is going to go bust if we don't learn to conserve. As the bible says, there is a season for all things. It is sometimes the season to say "no" more. Get one secondopinion if you do not agree with a doctor telling you enough is enough. However, at a certain point, enough *is* enough. This is why many doctors like to go to third world countries to practice. People are so grateful for any help. Many die without the luxuries we have, and it is just accepted as a way of life. Never forget how lucky we are to have such an amazing healthcare system, even when they do not give all you want. Sorry if I sound like I am preaching, but I do feel this personal entitlement is a factor in how we as a society continue to prolong the dying process. Just because it exists doesn't mean we should have it.

This was a very hard and emotionally draining chapter to write. I put out every emotional or coping skills reason why someone would hold on too long. I think it is pretty exhaustive. All my vulnerability with my own issues will be totally worth the effort if it just helps just one love nugget die with more peace in their hearts. If it helps anyone to mend their "dramas" or mend broken ties before it's too late. If one son or daughter could just closely examine a relationship before someone loses the mental ability to do so from dementia. If it just prevents at least one patient from physically suffering as their family was finally able to let them go sooner. I just want less suffering.

As you can see, I learned a lot from my mother, both good and bad. I feel the biggest lesson I learned was not to waste time and be fearless when dealing with emotional issues. If we can live fearless, then we can achieve inner peace. This peace would maybe change our death experience. How amazing would it be to die without fear? Then death can possibly be more of a celebration of the works of an amazing life, not result in years of sadness and regrets for those left behind. We can also possibly let go of trying to control death, as it is really beyond our human abilities. We can only focus on how we choose to live life.

Many do not like the fact I mention dementia is a terminal illness. I understand they feel persons with dementia will be dehumanized or objectified as symptoms and "interventions" and not people. The importance for me of mentioning how dementia is terminal is only to prevent some degree of suffering as people are dying. It is not to make people feel depressed or hopeless who have the illness. If anything, the awareness of how short life is, is a powerful motivator to finally live. I think every day what I will be like if I develop dementia. Again, I feel part of how I deal with dementia will be determined by how I lived life before dementia. With or without dementia, life itself is a terminal condition. A word should not scare you. My mother knew she had a terminal illness, and still accomplished a great deal. She did more living after hearing about her cancer.

I would like to end this chapter with a quote from Sogyal Rinpoche, the world-famous Tibetan Buddhist lama. "Normally we do not like to think about death. We would rather think about life. Why reflect on death? When you start to prepare for death you soon realize that you must look into your life now ... and come to face the truth of yourself. Death is like a mirror in which the true meaning of life is reflected."

CHAPTER 9

How to Choose a Nursing Home

➤ Find a home that doesn't have constant staff turnovers.

➤ Does the staff respond to call bells in a timely fashion.

➤ Does the home have a desk receptionist?

➤ Check the "nursing home state survey report."

➤ What activities are offered?

➤ Pick your battles carefully.

➤ Don't let *Best* become the enemy of the *Good Enough*.

The last two chapters were pretty tough. If you survived, I promise it will get lighter. I have really tried to avoid writing this next chapter. I was actually guilted into it by my editor. I don't think she meant to make me feel guilty, but it's really not that hard to do. I did consider cutting a zero out of the amount on her check for that extra stress. Then I thought about it and knew she was right. She phrased it in a way I could not resist. She told me about her mother, who became very ill in her nineties. She had to eventually find a nursing home to care for her. She said, "I was looking for a place where my mother would have to go to die." Well then, that's a whole different way to view the process. Let's just add that zero back and reconsider your idea. I really did need to write an opinion. I mean, I have wandered the halls of these places for twenty or more years—I should have an opinion. She made me realize how very important the issue is for people. No one would want their mother to die in a horrible place. I decided I was going to do my best to explain what I feel is a good nursing home.

What I Learned Early in My Career: Teamwork Works Best

I think I was avoiding discussing the issue for several reasons. Early on in my career I found myself starting to hate nursing homes. I was getting sick of walking into them. I resigned from ten of the twelve of them. I found them to be impossible places to work. I would see poor care a great deal of the time. I was also very young and idealistic when I started. I was going to help change their lives! If I had to write a letter to my younger self, I would say the following: "Dear Karen, you look pretty good in that new white coat. Damn, you are a doctor now! I hate to tell you, but it apparently is not so special anymore. People have Google, they don't need you. Sure you thought you were going to improve care, but you are just a small cog in the giant wheel of the way homes work. You are there so they can check that box that your evaluation is done. Don't annoy them with ideas and concerns about how to improve care. Suck it up and collect that paycheck girl, and go on with your bad self."

Ah, my life would be so much easier if I knew these facts back then. If I could just have overlooked care that bothered me and collected my paycheck like the others. My mother should have warned me about this aspect of the real world. She taught me to tell it like it is and stand up for what you believe. The keep-quiet-and-do-your-work route was never discussed. With her blunt approach, I would never have a job from what I can see now. Now that I think of it, her blunt style caused a bit of a scene in our neighborhood. One day, one of my mother's friends and neighbor came screaming into our yard. She had one of my mother's paintings that my mother had given to her nailed to a stick. She then proceeded to smash it on a tree in our yard. I assume my mother had told her something pretty bluntly. There goes mom, pissing off the neighbors again. I think you get where I am going with this example: in nursing homes, you can't complain too much about the care. If you notice a person crying in a dirty diaper, you try to discreetly get a staff member's attention. You don't make too big a fuss or you will be labeled that annoying doctor that points out our faults. You will be avoided. Eventually, if you point out their issues enough, you would *not* be asked back to provide care. The next thing you know, the consults will go to other doctors. Early in my career, I apparently did not follow that advice, and I paid for it. I was not shy about letting people in the administration know about bad care. I earned evil looks from nurses, nurses trying to sabotage my orders by calling other doctors to override me. Some would go online and make up bad reviews on those stupid doctor websites. As I was warned in med school, nurses will eat their own if you are on their bad side. You have to make the nurses happy, even the bad ones. Of course, there are some amazing nurses as well, as in all professions. Sadly, it only takes one or two bad ones to make life hell. I several times wanted to give up and leave all the homes. I then decided I had to stay and learn how to work the most efficiently in this unusual environment. They are systems you have to change in a gradual way, not with a hammer.

I just tried to make life easier for some elderly person. I bonded with the nurses who excelled, and we did what we could to improve care. I still work in two homes and have managed to work out good working relationships in these. We are more of a family than anything else. It is this kind of home that I want people to look for, the ones where you know the staff never changes. They do exist.

Nursing Home State Surveys

In preparation for this chapter, I did ask several of my more blunt friends how they would choose a home. One of my friends is the head nurse of nursing home; she is "smart," so I checked out her opinion. It was short and sweet, typical again for blunt people. She said to look at the nursing home state surveys posted online and in the homes.

"What are nursing home state surveys?" you might ask. Every year, the state surveys a home for a week. The surveyors sit at *all* the stations and watch *everything*. They pull out charts to explore for problems and talk to patients and their families for issues. For the staff, this is a week of hell. Surveyors never even smile to indicate how the staff is doing. The surveyors are tough.

I have seen many surveys. I have to say, there is no way that surveyors can catch all the stuff that goes on. I also noticed the homes totally change for the survey week. Everybody is on their best behavior. Each home has a survey window, so the staff knows approximately when they will be inspected. They go on overdrive to prepare. They will make sure every head staff is making rounds daily. They make sure patients have clean clothes. They respond to resident complaints and handle them immediately. The managers are answering call bells when they normally do not. None of the managers can get their administrative paper work done until the survey is over. Guess what! After the survey is over, everyone relaxes. The survey process never seemed fair or even helpful to me for this reason. Why should the homes have a notice when the surveyors are going to arrive! Surveyors need to drop in to see what happens everyday! What's this with "heads up?" I think you get my point about the surveys. They are useful, but their reports are not the main criteria by which I would pick a home for grandma.

There are other reasons surveys are unfair. There was one surveyor that was a big flirt. Every time he came to the building, there had to be one staff member to show cleavage. I think that's totally unfair. What if one home did not have the cleavage girl. Maybe they are all flat chested? Yes, this is very sexist. All joking aside, if you go to all the homes and asked, they would all be able to name this guy. Despite his eye for the ladies, he was actually a good surveyor. Maybe he has a neck condition and has trouble looking up?

The surveyors will look for problems and assign "tags." There are mild tags and serious tags depending on the actual issue. Tags are alphabet letters that are assigned to indicate a failing in the home. Just a note about the worst of the "tags" that can be given to a home. The bad tag is a G or IJ ("immediate jeopardy"). Those evaluations usually mean a monetary fine for the home. Furthermore, after a bad evaluation, the home may have to stop admitting new residents. I have seen one IJ tag. It was given to a home after a resident with an open wound on his foot had been smoking outside. Yes, some flies found the wound and then the maggots came. That resulted in an obvious IJ tag. The G tag I experienced was from a home not monitoring smokers. One smoking resident wandered too close to some oxygen tanks. Clearly, an explosion is not a good way to advertise your home, but will get you noticed!

Smokers are actually a hated part of the home; they cause too much liability. Nothing is more stressful than having a resident take a pain pill then going out to relax with a cigarette. It's bad publicity as well to have a resident catch on fire. No! Believe me it could really happen! If I could have a dollar for every cigarette burn in resident's clothes I have seen, I would be rich.

So how do nursing homes try to avoid these negative tags? I have heard several times that the head staff fabricated medical records. It's a rumor that passes around the building. Alarmingly, I have heard it more than once. Now that records are electronic, this may help stop this abuse. Altering medical records is about as low as a nursing home can drop in my opinion.

The nursing homes have to post their survey results in a readily available location. Most times I see them on a stand in the front entrance. Their scoring is fully explained in the Medicare website called "Nursing Home Compare." The Medicare website contains a great deal of information on nursing homes and is very much worth your time. Just because I say homes know how to skirt around getting tags, does not mean that the ratings have no value. I feel that surveyors should exclude homes that perform poorly but not throw out homes that have some issues. These tags are one part of a whole picture. I would read through each tag and see if it is a minor tag. Sometimes, the home was also just unlucky and got a really tough surveyor.

The Call Bell Problem

The biggest complaint I hear from residents is that the staff is not answering the call bells in a timely manner. The residents squeeze a bulb that turns on a light in the hallway. The nurse has to come in and shut it off manually and find out what the resident needs. Apparently, the aides have to answer all call bells in ten minutes or so. The biggest complaint I receive from residents is about the call bells. I even see the surveyors themselves ringing the bells to time how fast they respond. I hate to say it, but I too have tested the aides as well. Every time a resident complained to me about their aide being slow, I would test the bell in front of them. I have to say I never caught an aide being late. But I am sure a few aides have silently cursed me.

Sometimes, the call bells also make a buzzing noise at the nursing station to alert nurses in addition to the light. It's a sound that would make me want to stab a pencil in my ear to stop the annoying pain. Sometimes passersby ask us, "How can you stand that sound!" Ignoring the call bell is apparently a skill the nurses learn quickly. In psychiatry, we call that dissociation. It is a way to deal with a traumatic situation. For example, it is similar to when you are driving in your car and you suddenly arrive at your destination not recalling the drive. It's all a big blur, and you think, "How did I get here?" Well, I assume it's the same process that happens when the nurses are on their shifts. The call bells become that noise in the background. I imagine it's a survival tool as the nurses have to pass out meds, direct the aides, write notes, answer phone calls, and answer passersby questions. If you do not tune out a little, you may lose your mind. After all, the homes no longer seem to pay for a desk receptionist, and nurses are doing more and more with less and less. You know a place cares when the home hires a desk clerk in the day to assist the nurses. I feel it should be mandatory.

Sundowning

The night shift is a whole new world. It's the time when the sundowners get going. A common occurrence in dementia cases, with sundowning, the patient typically experiences a period of confusion later in the day and into the night. The staff is stretched even more so at these times as residents become increasingly anxious and difficult to control. During this part of the day, the call bells are answered even slower. It is more possible then, more than any other time of the day, the nurse shuts off the call bell and says, "I will be right back." Oh yeah, you are in trouble then. You are probably sitting there wondering what "right back" means for the next twenty minutes. I have no good advice on that one. It basically means the aid will be back when they are done with all their other chores. In all fairness to the nurses, there is the confused call bell ringer who sets it off constantly. They are ringing that darned bell every five minutes. Such residents, of course, may have a short-term memory span of say three minutes. You guessed it; after the three minutes have passed they ring the bell again as if it was the first time. They forget it was answered, and the next day they tell me they waited two hours for the nurses to answer their bell. I will generally find their call bell tied behind the bed or on the floor so they have to stop ringing. Another option is for the nurses to hide the bell is to slide it into the crevice of the mattress. Eventually, the resident may even call the nurse's station from the phone. The best is when they decide to call 911 to get help. I know it's hard to believe, but it happens all the time. I would love to be a police officer on the other end of that phone call when the emergency is "need to be changed."

Regardless, the call bell is the biggest issue I hear about from patients. If you are deciding on a home, stand in the hallway and just watch to see how long it takes for the bells to get answered. Hopefully the home will allow it. You need to make sure you drop in to look at a home at both day and night.

Activities

Other features that I look for are the level of activities. I hate to say it, but most homes do the "plant and go." They "plant" the resident around a television and "go" do their work. It's usually a game show on the TV. There have been times I have gone to facilities to hear music playing as they are planted. Sometimes it is age appropriate music. But then there are those times that the hip-hop is on. I particularly love those times the hip-hop is on and nurses are asking me to medicate the patients for agitation. I think you can follow what I am saying. I would advise you pay attention to what is on the televisions as they offer a secret signal to whom the staff is most interested in entertaining: themselves or the residents.

My favorite home actually had activities all day long. I have never seen anything like it before and never have since. It was a smaller home of course—about ninety beds. The activity director's name is Nicole from West Palm Beach. She is amazing and it was a wonderful uplifting atmosphere going on in there. We have to recognize star staff if we want our homes to excel. If you can guess who it is I am talking about, call her and offer her a lot of money to come to your home. She kept those brain's buzzing. I saw a lot of trivia and reminiscing. You could never be bored in this place. The level of activity in a home is really crucial. You can ask for a calendar of events for the residents when you walk in the home. I would take a close look at it: there is a lot of time in a day to fill. I feel this should be one of the strongest aspects of a home. Homes should also try to gear the activities to the individual patients. I personally would be sick of constant bingo. The men in the homes hate bingo. Every now and then I will see a place get a good card game going with the men and the ladies. I feel gambling is a totally awesome idea in the homes. Let's be fair to our seniors. After all, their last concern is a gambling addiction.

I have to make one point about activities to be fair to the nursing homes. One thing that did drive the staff crazy was the families who insisted that their parent be forced into the activity room. It's one of those questions you have to do a double take when you hear it. You are imaging in your head how you force someone into a room. I suppose if you tip a wheelchair backward and roll them in the room, they could not say no. I was then told chair tipping was not allowed! We could try telling several lies to get them in, like strippers for the men and foot rubs for the ladies. That scenario would result in a mass exit of an angry elderly mob, once they caught on to the lie. Like my three year old tells me, "That's just not cool." Homes can't force people into activities, no matter how exciting the activity. They can't force anyone to do anything.

Food

I am going to make this one paragraph short. All nursing home food is kinda gross at some point. Making mass produced food is never easy. Please bring your parents food from home as much as possible. Thank you ahead of time.

Staff Turnover

As an insider, I have a few other thoughts on nursing homes. I would look at staff turnover. The homes that have the same staff forever and ever, combined with good inspection reports, are the best. It generally means there is a team working together. Nursing home care is a team approach, and it starts with the administrator. The best homes I work in have had the same staff forever, and we feel like family. I think this is a great way to inspect a home. You are, after all, going to have to build very close relationships with these people. They will be getting to know all the intimate information about you and your family. Ask to speak to the charge nurse, make sure she has people skills. Too often, the tour guides do not let you stop and get to know the staff. Be sneaky, as your family member's future depends on it. Again, drop in at different times of the day. You can try to pull staff or even other families aside and get to know the real deal.

Certified Nurses' Assistants

I often wonder what else I would do to ensure my loved one's happiness. I think what it all comes down to is that certified nurses' assistants (CNA) are the backbones of good care. I have the utmost respect for them, as no one really knows what they go through. In Florida, they are mainly Jamaican and Haitian. One home I know in Maryland has staff from Senegal. Don't be put off by your prejudices. Often in poorer cultures or in non-Western cultures, people in general have more respect for the elderly. In the Maryland home, respect for elders is automatically built into Senegalese culture. These African workers treat their patients with tenderness and great care plus lots of joking along the way. Certified nursing assistants earn very low salaries for the type of work they perform. It is backbreaking lifting much of the time. I feel horrible when I hear how they are spoken to at times. Racism is alive and well in the elderly. I lost track of how many times I have heard the "N" word. The aides must somehow have to keep trying to block all that out. They are hit and kicked at all the time. How do you maintain your morale in that position? CNA's can be understaffed and be tortured by families and nurses if there are too many call bells. I can see if they could become angry and even at risk for losing their tempers. To be honest, they should make much higher pay and be made to feel a part of the team. I have always for that reason tried to say hello to them in passing. I ask them their opinions on the resident's behaviors. With all the nurses having to spend more time documenting in the charts, the aides are the ones who really know what is going on. If my mother were in the home, I would totally treat her CNA like family. I have always believed what my mother would say, "you get more with sugar than vinegar." I can't emphasize this enough. The CNA are going to be your family. I don't care if you are in a million dollar home, or a three-star forty-year-old building. The staff that provides the most direct care is the one I care about most. And that person is usually the certified nursing assistant.

Crime, Drugs, Alcohol

Other tips: be careful of the crime in the area. I had one home in a bad area next to a convenience store. The next thing I know, a woman tipped her electric wheelchair over while drunk. I guess those scooters don't go up curbs well. Then we later found a resident selling pot to the other residents in dime bags. It's amazing how many different ways you can supplement your social security income.

The Sniff Test

I often get asked about smells in home. I wish this were a good way to judge a home. I hate to break this to everyone, but poop smells bad. It's really hard to change a Depends and keep the smell in the room. I have walked down the hallways and past rooms where I thought I would die a slow death due to the smell. I would not judge any home on this, more so the overall smell. I suppose if the home generally reeks of urine, then that's a really bad sign. I have rarely been in a home that had that bad of a urine smell. The one place I did was actually an assisted living facility. I realized they were dealing with the issue by putting down strong bleach products. Bleach is a cheap way to hide the smell. Ever since then, I avoid places that have that strong bleach smell. I figure they are so cheap that instead of putting down new floors, they spill cheap cleaners on them. Carpets are obviously a bad idea in homes. The smell stays forever. Most homes seem to be turning to hardwood floors. Generally, the older a home, the more smells you will get. I don't have a great answer on smells. Overall, it is not one of the major issues. Several of my homes pull out the bread-making machine when the state survey is expected. They at least smell great for that week.

Who Is There Looking After Grandma?

A few other bonuses to look for in the homes: do they employ full time nurse practitioners and/or a full time medical director? If so, you will have a medical professional around at all times. This is very valuable for your loved one. At some homes, they just have a private doctor who contracts to visit weekly. They are the building's medical director. They collect a monthly stipend to see patients and direct care. I have to be honest. I have worked with some real duds of doctors in the homes. We all know they do "drive by" rounds. They peek in the door to see if the patients are breathing. They speak to the nurse and write the same redundant note in the chart. They can get away with it because the patients are confused. I hold my breath when an alert patient catches them. Once a man approached me asking why he had a bill from this doctor was supposedly seeing him monthly. He said he had not seen the doctor for months. I mean, the answer was really obvious, but you don't want to say, "Because your doctor is committing Medicare fraud and ripping you off! I hate those awkward moments. I just told him he could call the number on the bill if he had any questions. The same doctor writes the same note on the same patient every time. I would read his notes and think they were really cut and paste. The home knew, as I would tell them, but at least they had a medical director. There are not many doctors who want to work in homes, so there is little the homes can do. They "take what they can get" to meet residents needs. I always prefer the doctors who send ARNP's or a PA as they are more accessible for questions. Lastly, the doctors that round extremely early or past 9pm are not ideal as well. They maybe, not always are trying to get away with the drive by rounds on residents.

There maybe a few other brave doctors who will come to nursing homes. These doctors will only go on staff if they are guaranteed several patients to make it worth their while. Your personal doctor will not be there. Nursing homes will not let any doctor in who is not fully credentialed to write orders in their building. However, homes are more likely to let a doctor in if the doctor provides them patient referrals. Homes do try to find quality doctors, but of course they want to know what the doctor can bring to the table. I have witnessed these discussions several times. I have been expected to refer patients in order to be allowed in the home. All I personally can offer is psychiatric care. It's a tricky path to follow, as we have the "Stark Laws" in Florida. Our medical school faculty never taught us about the Stark Laws. I had to learn on the job. They are the anti-kickback laws. We are not allowed to get kickbacks or benefits for any patient referrals. This law does not stop people from trying. The combination to be aware of is a doctor who works for a nursing home and a home health company. This just screams possible inappropriate referrals.

When I first moved to Florida, the home health companies and pharmaceutical companies were full force. These companies always wanted to throw parties for the doctors and take us out for drinks. They wanted the doctors to send the discharged patients home with their company or use their medications. I was told it was the Wild West, and it was true. The nursing homes gave out the referrals based on the number of referrals the home health companies would give to them. By law, nursing homes have to offer a choice. You think that you have a choice of the company when you are leaving. In reality, the choice is the company the home knows and is getting the most from. I was so turned off that I avoided all those companies. It took me a minute to figure it out, but then I realized home health companies didn't like to spend time with me because of my glowing personality: they saw me as a dollar sign. I dropped all contact with them. I was fine being hated. It was actually a compliment.

The same issues of one hand greasing another can happen when your parent ends up with the broken hip in the hospital. It's an unexpected emergency no one really prepares to face. The case managers will approach your room and inform you that you need to pick a nursing home to finish the rehabilitation process. This is when you want to throw up your hands, as everything you have heard about these homes is horrible. You have a day or two to figure it out—an impossible task. The case managers have a lot of pressure on them to get the discharges done, as the insurance companies will stop paying if the discharges take too long. The case managers also have to deal with families who want to take their time to research a place. If that is not enough, the family is also bombarded by marketers from the nursing homes showing their products. "Pick me, pick me," I imagine them saying. The marketers visit with candy and cakes and smiles. They want the business. Somehow, the hospital case manager may come up with a list of places they prefer to send the patients. Most of them have never even stepped foot in these places. They can only rely on the marketing and word of mouth. I honestly do not understand the full process of how a home is chosen. I know the type of insurance the patient holds plays a part. Humana, for instance, only approves a limited number of homes. If you have Medicare, the world is your oyster. The homes love straight Medicare with a secondary insurance. They are the best payer source. The home may even drool on you as you come through the door. Relying on a hospital caseworker is not the best choice, despite their good intentions. I recommend you look at these homes right after the crisis of the broken hip occurs, and not wait till you get the call for discharge.

There is one other really odd issue that prevents discharge from the hospital. It's not even the families. There are homes that actually run away from certain types of patients and families. The nursing homes shop for potential patients on the Internet as well as from calls they receive from case managers. A few times a month, they ask me to review the prospects. Why me? Because no home wants the patients with the psych issues, especially those with violent behaviors. They want the orthopedic patients. The patients with serious wounds are avoided as well; the home doesn't want to be blamed for not being able to cure a wound. If a patient has to be on a ventilator and dialysis at the same time, the care is too expensive for the home to make a profit. If the home feels the expectations for success are low and the family expectations for success are too high, this sets up the concerns for potential lawsuits. The homes will tend to take more of these patients they dislike when the census is low. The more popular homes can be even pickier. If you want to get into them, you need to downplay any psychiatric issues. It's a sad reality, but I have seen it over and again.

Conclusion: Don't Let the "Best" Be the Enemy of the "Good Enough"

I hope I have not depressed you all from the search. I just want to let you know what goes on behind the scenes in nursing homes. Finding a nursing home that's "best" is impossible. Finding a "good enough" nursing home is a lot easier. I have created a checklist to summarize all these considerations:

1. Research "Nursing Home Compare" at the Medicare website.

2. Schedule a visit to the home, but try to spend time there without the marketer present. Talk to the aides and the unit managers about staff turnover, length at the job. They will be unlikely tell you the "dirt," but what the heck, it's worth a try.

3. Watch the call bells by looking at the lights on the doors. See how fast they are answered.

4. Visit later in day, after 5 p.m. when the big chiefs are not there.

5. Look for carpet stains, damaged walls, and anything that looks run down. If the home is not willing to reinvest in repairs, that is not a good sign.

6. Look the activity lists. If they only have a few activities per day, then how are residents entertained in between? Are they planted in front of a television? If they are planted, are the staff involved with them? Many times, there is someone sitting there and not attempting to interact or engage with the residents.

7. Look at what activities are available for men. The men are often overlooked. No man really wants a mani and pedicure that I have ever met.

8. Find out who will be the doctor assigned. It is always better if they have a nurse practitioner that rounds with and for them. This will give you more access to ask questions.

9. Find out how long the administrator and director of nurses have held the job. If every few years there is a change, that is a sign the building maybe struggling to find order.

10. Ask how psychiatric issues will be managed, especially if someone becomes aggressive. Will they be committed to a psychiatric hospital if they hit other patients? All people with dementia can eventually become aggressive, so this question should always be asked. If you do not want them ever committed, be prepared for psychiatric medications to be used.

The Personal Touch

Once you find your home, decorate, decorate, decorate. Make it warm and full of love. You are going to be a big part of what makes it a great experience. Also, pick and choose your battles with the home. One social worker told me to not complain about every little issue; then you will have less weight with the big issues. Staff will run for cover when they see the constant complainer walk in the home. As I have told you in my own experience with complaining about poor care, there is a way to do it to get the best result. Over-all, remember they DO want to make your experience a good one. Yelling and belittling the staff when they do not live up to your image of a good home solves nothing. Over and over I see families try this out of frustration, not all families, but some.. It solves nothing and makes staff avoid you. I know it's hard to think your loved one maybe suffering because of bad care, but deal with your frustration in other ways. Bond with the staff and they will go over and above for you. I have seen many aides become family, sit and chat with your family members when you are not there. They go above and beyond when they are treated kindly. All nurses went into the field to help others. Learn how to unlock their full potentials with positivity and appreciation. It will go a long way to a good experience.

CHAPTER 10

Advice for the Baby Boomer

After spending so much time in nursing homes, I started planning more for my own slow demise. Yes, we all hope we just die in our sleep, but I prepare for both a sudden and a slow death. I am sure that sounds morbid, but I have no issues with it. I am one of the baby boomers, ready to pass into the over 65 range. I was never a boy scout, but I am totally prepared. So how does when get to the point where you are preparing so much younger? I supposed it is from seeing others age and die so often. Once you see all the ways you can die, you are a much better planner.

I do try to keep my body healthy. After a year of doing autopsies, I still recall what cholesterol looks like in your arteries. I try not to eat "crap food," but I do break down weekly and treat myself. I figure if I exercise, it will blow out the old pipes and counteract the fat load from the fries. Overall, I am a decent eater. I go to the doctor yearly and take their advice. If there are things I can do to increase my chance of living longer, then why not? I don't go crazy with it, but I don't avoid it due to fear of what the doctor will find. I like my body, and I want it to be happy. It has done a lot for me.

I have to say, being a doctor makes you more paranoid about your health. I recall back to medical school, we all thought we had the disease we were reading about for the week. The term for this phenomenon is called the "medical student disease." For a year, I was getting migraines and was convinced that I had a brain aneurysm. I somehow talked a doctor into getting an MRI. Actually, I knew how to get doctors to order the tests I wanted. I could easily make a story close to what a doctor would worry about, then say, "I hope I don't have a brain aneurysm." I know how they think, once you suggest it then they have to rule it out. No matter what anyone says, as doctors we still think there is a lawyer behind every patient giving legal advice. I have been laughing lately at the new billboards in Palm Beach from lawyers. They post this corny picture of some woman smiling with a handful of cash saying, "So and so lawyer just got me one million dollars." I was imagining the poor fools life she ruined with stress so she could slather Ben Franklin's all over her body on a public billboard. Well, I used that fear to get my MRI. I never ended up having an aneurysm. I supposed I had the reassurance I was not dying, at least not from an aneurysm.

Besides keeping your body tuned up, there is a lot of paperwork you have to do to prepare for the end. I am still not sure where and how I want to be buried. It's such a hard decision. Caskets kind of creep me out. I could be cremated, but then I become more like a dust collector on a shelf. I have always hated clutter. I suppose people could split me up and each keep a dust pile of me. I think I would rather be sprinkled in a Japanese garden we have here in Florida. At least my family could enjoy some good sake and sushi when they visited my essence there. I am not sure what I would be called, an essence or a spirit, something that sounds profound I supposed. The garden is a peaceful place and relaxing, I will consider the idea.

I knew I had to do some other preparation before I kick the bucket. All this paperwork is a pain but we have to do it. I did the power of attorney papers and all the other legal work I needed to protect my family. I had seen way too many younger people become ill and not be prepared. I am still shocked at how little people really understand power of attorney papers. I have heard hundreds of times from people "I am my own power or attorney, I don't need one." Nope, you can't be your own power of attorney, as it is impossible. The more I have had to explain it, the more blunt I become. "Say, if you get hit by a car and you are unconscious and can't talk, maybe on a machine. Who will talk to the doctors for you and who will pay your bills." Quick and dirty usually gets the job done. Who do you trust to make your medical and financial decisions should you be unable to make your own? That sounds more doctorly. Trust me, do it early. Many times, people sneak in lawyers in the homes to get people to sign things. They may be completely confused and have no idea what they are signing. If you like all your hard earned savings to be used properly, get your papers done. If not, they may fall into the hands of that annoying cousin or sibling you have secretly hated.

Living wills also have to be completed. Do you want to be resuscitated if your heart stops? Oh yes, do you want tubes to be kept in if you have no chance at a meaningful life? Sadly, I have also seen people's living wills overturned by the power of attorney (POA). Apparently, everyone has a different opinion of what a meaningful life looks like. You really need to discuss this with whom you choose to be your POA. I hate to tell people this, but even after all this paperwork; people may still go against your wishes. I did not think it was possible, until I saw it happen. People who never wanted to live on tubes, stay on tubes. I think it happens most often when the POA does not want to believe the doctor on the prognosis. I have seen several doctors tell this one family that there was no chance of improvement. The family insisted there was a chance and refused hospice. Hey, I am the first one who loves a miracle. If one happens then awesome, but my motto has always been, hope for the best, and plan for the worst. If the best happens while you are planning for the worst, then you are having an awesome day. The man I am referring to did finally pass away as they were waiting for that miracle. If several people are telling you there is no chance for improvement, they are generally right. If it were just one, then I would get a consensus. Either way, don't let someone suffer as you are trying to decide. A lot can happen with your original will, so grill your POA well. I have grilled my POA and made sure they do not succumb to guilt or fear of losing me as a motivating factor to keep my tubes. You let me suffer, and I will make you suffer in the next life.

There is one factor that people rarely consider, how afraid your doctor is that you will sue for a bad outcome. There are still some doctors (who see that same billboard of the lawsuit-happy lady) who will bend your POA papers. They are so afraid to be honest with families that they do whatever is asked, no matter how unreasonable. I had one patient insist we have a brain CT scan of her clearly demented husband. Many doctors just do as they are asked to avoid the confrontation and the lawsuit. I told her that we were not doing any tests that were not going to help us. A CT scan was not going to change our treatment of him. I, of course, was not very popular and not asked to come back. I refuse to be the doctor that does what a family wants, just because they want it. I have heard countless nurses complain about that doctor who "just does everything the family says," no matter how unrealistic. I am thinking this is the kind of doctor who may not follow your last wishes?

You may want to ask your primary care doctor to follow your wishes in front of your POA. Just a thought. Maybe I am paranoid at this point, but I want to hear my doctor will be strong in the face of my pressuring family. I do understand the doctors who want to keep their sanity by just agreeing. It is a much smoother ride as a doctor. I just disagree with those doctors. I feel we are obligated to be truthful, even if it upsets people.

Once you have the papers completed, you are pretty much set. If you are older and into your 60s, you may want to look at possible places you can retire. Places that can assist you should you develop a medical illness. A place you can go in an emergency. Just at least drive by some places, get costs and look at their surveys. You can even ask around. People always wait until it is an emergency and then look.

If you are starting to be concerned about your aging parents, then you should scope out places for them. Don't wait for an emergency! I keep repeating not to wait because we see so many people who wait for an emergency. You can even have an emergency folder with all the important information ready to go. All the medical, legal, and financial papers in your little hot hand. You will have to bring it to each new place. Just because you gave it to the hospital, doesn't mean the hospital gave it to the nursing home. You will have to fill out whether you have a living will or not, do you want to have CPR, etc. all over again.

There is one more aspect to prepare for, as we all get ready to push up some daisies. How are we going to prepare for retirement? Working with all ages more recently, I have realized one thing. You have to have hobbies. Not just any hobby, ones that can be done with little physical activity. What would you do if you could not play tennis, golf, or swim any longer? Can you watch a lot of television? Hope you like to read, as you will have lots of time. I am thinking there will be much more electronics than there are now. More video games for sure, I am hoping, as this is a nice alternative. So few are Internet savvy in the generation in nursing homes now. Learn about computers! I probably will be doing what I do best—goofing off. As long as I can be around people, I am hoping I will be all right. I will probably volunteer when I can't play sports. Hobbies are just something to keep in mind, as retirement is a challenging period.

We also have to mentally prepare for a potential loss of independence. This can be the most difficult part of aging. Can you handle someone wiping your tush? How about giving you a shower or bed bath? I am not sure about you, but pretty sure this will suck. I am very modest. I have to think that they have seen every type of boob and butt and mine are not somehow different. You may also have to give up your finances to someone else to do. Some have to sell their cars. Just be ready in your head that anything is possible. Again, hope for the best and plan for the worst. It will make it easier on your children as well.

If you do end up in a home, how would you want it decorated? What of your personal belongings would you want with you? So many people who move to nursing homes unexpectedly, wanted that chance to go through their belongings and pick and choose what they want. "I want to go through my stuff by myself and pick out what I want!" I have heard that so many times, but that is an impossible request sometimes. Why not tell your family what belongings you want to keep before that time comes? Of course, there is always someone who can't get over having to let go of their belongings. They want everything. You can't put all your value in your belongings. I am not me unless I have my "stuff." For me it is different; I don't get attached to objects. I realize others are not the same way, so I try not to judge. I just know it's impossible to take it all with you. The most I would like are pictures of my family, maybe some nice pictures on my walls of nature. If I can't take it with me when I cash in my chips, it doesn't have any value for me. My mother always reminded me, "build your treasures in heaven".

This is a good lead into my final paragraph. We talked about body, and legal papers, and now the most important, the spiritual. I have never been religious; I have been spiritual. The difference for me is the guilt. Religion always made me somehow feel guilty and just wrong. I connected more with spiritual, as it was more uplifting for me. I felt God was the purest form of love we can attain. God is love and vice versa. This is all I need to know; it is what I spend my life trying to figure out. How can I get to the purest form of love for others and myself? It really is a daily task. It involves talking to yourself with the language of love. And all else follows. The more we like ourselves, the more we like others, the less judgmental and angry we become. I read a book many years ago; yes it was a long time ago because my attention deficit does not permit me to read much. It was called the Celestine Prophecy. What impacted me about it was how we are made of energy. If you study energy, you know it has different levels of vibration. I feel love has an energy. The more unconditional and positive it is, the stronger its vibration. It is contagious to others. They feel better being around you and taking a hit off your energy. I now try to surround myself with people who have positive energy. The negative people keep sucking my energy, and it gets pretty annoying. Anyone who complains, is bitter, blames others, holds on to anger, puts down people, I avoid them like the plague. For me, they are a contagious illness. No one steals my energy. I feel that negative energy harms your immune system and helps diseases to grow. What ever I can do to get rid of the negative, I am on it. For years I was angry with my mother and father; I went to therapy and dealt with it. Why carry that crap around—it's only hurting you. I am always practicing these things; one day I will be really good at it. Speaking of energy, I now tell people who feel there is nothing after death one thing, "energy can neither be created or destroyed, only rearranged." Take that one, chew on it a while. We have no choice but to go somewhere per this law. Be prepared. I assume it will be levels of energy we can't even imagine possible. One big energy meatball in the sky! Well, just a theory.

We can love ourselves, but we are also trying to love others deeply. This is for me one other preparation for the aging process. What relationships you develop in your life and how deeply you can love, are to me the real treasures. As I have said, our belongings are not what bring us happiness in the end. We all struggle to have the nicest house, the biggest bank account, and what matters the most is our relationships. We are so busy and "have so much to do today," that we again forget to connect with those around us. Everyday, I try to ask myself, "is there something I should have said to someone but I didn't?" Is there an anger I held in that is hurting me? I am nowhere near perfect, but I try my hardest to follow this path. In the end, when we have nothing else, those who love us are the most important. How we loved will be the most important memory we leave behind. How we loved will be carried by our children and their children. It is a gift that will transcend time. Don't waste years before you try to learn this lesson. Our children will be sad to see us leave, but they will have this gift forever. It will give them confidence to be strong and loving people as well.

I also let my children know that I can care for myself in all aspects. I love having them in my life, but they are not responsible for me. Whatever is supposed to happen to me is my path and journey, it was meant to be and my destiny. There is no place for them to feel guilty or responsible. I will be ready to let go when my time is near.

If they want to tell me it is okay to leave them, that would make me feel better, but I will be fine either way.

The last thing I have taught them is the one that has helped me the most, the ability to play. Never be afraid to be that child, goofy, silly, and free. Splash in the rain, run in puddles, smear pudding on your face, and laugh. Fart and blame it on the dog. Pick your nose and pretend to eat it. Just laugh as if you do not care. Before I die, I would love to do what we did as kids. Burp and ask your sister what it tasted like. Not caring about what anyone thinks or says about you is the ultimate freedom. When I get to this point, I think I would also have no fear of death, and that nothing will change who am. Neither death, illness or any other external factor.

CHAPTER 11

Happy Endings

That Special Massage?

My editor Helen persuaded me to write about "Happy Endings." She had to clarify that it was not a chapter that was going to contain older naked men and a massage table. Nor was it a steamy romance story about late life love. It's about the residents I did treat who actually did well in the homes. They had a QQ equation that was definitely a good quality of life, despite the unknown quantity left. I don't want to leave my readers with a terrible view of nursing homes. There are some success stories! I have worked my career trying to get more of these stories and less of the suffering I witnessed. Many times, success was a painless, peaceful passing to the next world. Success comes in many forms.

In writing this chapter, I decided to ask all the patients I see (who could have a conversation) what they would want to make them happy. It was actually an amazing experience as I learned some new things about the elderly. I was a little afraid to ask the question at first. I thought I would get the long list of how they hate mystery meat or the wait for the aides. I even pressed a few people because they had no complaints. Are you sure? Do you remember where you are? One woman, Esther, had been in the home quite a while. When I first started working with her, she very depressed and suffering in pain. It was hard to visit and see her so sad, I felt at times I had failed her. I know it's an irrational thought, but it was there and I accepted it. Today was different; she told me she was very content! This is a woman who never leaves her bed or her room if at all possible. I could not understand how she could be content in this situation. "I just need a good book and a little television," she said. Of course, I wondered how long she had been reading the same book, but it didn't matter as it made her happy. I guess the antidepressants didn't hurt either. Just when I thought she was going to stay depressed forever, she proved me wrong. I was glad I had asked since part of me was starting to avoid her, as I could not fix her. I am sure I have many of the same feelings as do families, we are all human. It reminded me to continue to force myself into the sad situations as one day they may resolve.

Spaghetti

I moved to the next bed, a little old woman named Ruth. Her head is always kinked to the right, so I always talk to her with my head tilted the same direction. I suppose that makes no sense, as it doesn't help me hear better. I guess I feel more connected when I tilt my head? She usually complains to me all the time. I asked her the question and then sat in dread of the answer. I'm waiting for it, here it comes, it's going to be bad. "I would love some spaghetti and meatballs." Really? Are you for real? That's all you want? I told her I had no idea she was Italian. "No, I'm Jewish, but I am really craving spaghetti." All right, I get it; this Italian girl loves her meatballs too. Did her antidepressants work that well all the sudden? Who cares, she is happy today; don't question it. Then I started to realize that there was a certain type of resident who seemed to cope well with being in the homes. I hate to say it, but the people who are satisfied with the least, seemed to me the happiest. They needed so little and had low expectations. The ones who said, "If I just had this, or if I was just home, or if my kids would just visit more" always struggled. Do you have to give up the fight that you are going to leave, to finally be happy where you are? I guess a life lesson for us all. Once you stop fighting the fact that you have to cope with a situation, you can start coping with the situation.

The Raccoons

Let me follow with a few more success stories. I have a patient I followed for years, and I feel she has made me very happy. Her name is Betty. I loved her and still do. She was always in her wheelchair rolling around the facility, out on the smoking patio. I would say smoking was her hobby. She had married an older man who also lived in the home. His name was Milton. She would always make jokes about how they were having sex. I would think, "Sure you are Betty," and then I would wonder if it was really somehow possible. She would always kiss my cheek. I had to bend forward to her chair and my hair would always fall in her face. I would always apologize for my hair. She would then leave a little spit mark on me every single time she kissed me. I would take the wet glob like a real woman because I loved her. I knew it made her happy. She was also the resident council president in the home and always involved with some peer gossip. She did it in this raspy voice as her vocal cords were coated in tar and nicotine; it made it all the more funny. She hated this other woman there named Madge. Madge hated her as well. When they were mad at each other, they would have these awesome verbal altercations. I like the word altercation, sounds more psychiatric. They actually would even run against each other to be the Resident Council President. There were only a few people who were with it enough to vote, so I am not sure how either won. There was not a smoking area big enough for the both of them. I always dreaded when they were on the psych list after another fight. I do recall one fight over Madge's cat. Madge would feed the stray cats around the homes. She had this big fat black cat that walked with a limp that she called her pet. Every now and then, it would stray in the building to find Madge. It was so fat I wanted to offer it an insulin shot or maybe some physical therapy. Well, the chubby cat was not all that Madge attracted with the free food. One day, Madge attracted the raccoons to the patio with her food. As building president, Betty was not going to allow that! She went into action to block all feedings on the patio. It was the talk of the home. Don't worry; the black cat is still there waiting to have a coronary event, still hanging out in Madge's room. The raccoons are gone though.

Betty was not always happy and fun as she is now. When I first started there, she had her times when she was severely depressed and anxious. She would pace the hall and look for me each time I came to the building. After numerous medication changes, she was amazing. She even survived the death of Milton. It was a sad time, and it was hard to see his bed filled by another. I love just sitting with her on the smoking patio and listening to her talk crap about Madge. Sometimes, I get some good dirt about the staff as well. Betty is another resident who doesn't ask for much. She just loves to shoot the breeze and make inappropriate comments. She also just wanted love, and she gave it just as easily.

Breaking up the Drug Ring!

Madge was also pretty amazing in her own way. She could walk and probably didn't need to be in a nursing home, but she made it like a real home. She would wheel around in her chair and I would see her deliver mail from time to time. She was another who suffered bad depressions initially until the medications finally kicked in. She was also our facility gardener and actually built a tremendous garden around the smoking patio. She should have been paid for the work she did at this home. She even had butterfly gardens. She had a severe neck problem as well as a history of alcoholism. This caused the doctors a real dilemma, as they were always afraid she would abuse the medications. She was always fighting to get more pain meds until she kept ending up looking snookered a few times. Betty told us once that she fell forward out of her wheelchair while gardening. Guess she was a little buzzed on pain meds. She was even involved in a nursing Percocet ring once. A nurse was stealing narcotics from the residents. When she was caught, she snuck the little bag of her stash to Madge. Madge then hid the stash in a room with a confused woman. The guilt was too much and she confessed. What a woman, busting up a drug ring.

Things changed for her briefly when she was told her spinal bones were going to collapse around her spinal cord and she would become a paraplegic. I remember that day well: if something had stopped her from being able to garden then I am afraid her soul would let go. She was warned to take it easy. She asked me several times if I believed the doctors were correct. I told her that no one knows. She eventually stopped going to doctors and just kept gardening. I thought that would be the end to her spirit but no, she gardens to this day. Still no signs of paraplegia.She ignores the fear and goes on. Pretty amazing. She cusses like a sailor, another excellent quality that will prolong life. Screw your bad back, I am planting this flower. She could say that! I love that tough old broad.

A Dinner Date

The next story really impacted me a great deal. It started out sad and then became amazing for me. It was about a little old guy name Richard. He came into my home after his wife had just passed. He was a skinny little thing and only talked looking down. He was handling the death of his wife very poorly. He wanted to die as well and was not shy about telling people. It's always an awkward conversation when someone demands to die, and you tell them no. I mean, how far do you take the conversation. I finally tell people, "Listen, I can't kill you and you can't kill yourself so you just have to wait to die like the rest of us." I feel at times like its the same conversation I have when my kids want to get a present and it's not their birthday, except I tell them they can't get a present because they don't have a job to afford one. I generally did not argue with Richard. "Yes, Richard, I know you want to die, I understand." I promised the family I would give him an antidepressant to see if it changed him mood. They wanted him to live so badly as they had just lost their mother. I would pass by his room and talk to the son a few times. I overheard him once tell his father, "Listen Dad, I can't lose you. I just lost Mom, and I am not going to lose you now." This is not what Richard wanted to hear. The family wanted to press on with physical therapy and even talk of a tube for his stomach as he ate so poorly. One day, I went to the home to find Richard and see what how he was doing. The nurse relayed an interesting story to me. Richard told the nurse he was leaving that night to go have dinner with his wife. Shortly after this, he died. Yep, he left to go have dinner with his wife. How the heck he knew this was the case blows me away. I still always think of him up in heaven at a table, smiling at her as he shared a meal. He finally had what he wanted.

Anyone in Pants!

I have to share a few stories about my really confused residents. They get to be happy sometimes, even when they have advanced dementia. Thank God that dementia sometimes progresses to where you are happy because you do not understand the situation you are in now. We all loved those residents. It was part of the job we really enjoyed; things people would do would make us laugh. It was just like when my four-year-old would say something totally outrageous, and you laugh. What they say is true: you go out like you come into the world. No hair, no teeth, in diapers and you say the darnedest things. One woman named Ruth; she was so in love with men. It was not just one guy, it was all men. Talk about role reversals, she was always hot on the trail of anyone in pants with a package. She would start with one guy, and then see another. In a few minutes she would go to the new guy and ask if he was single and that he looked really good. By the end of the day, she had been with every guy in the building. Thankfully, none of them minded.

She eventually died of cancer, but she had a good time until the end. She flirted day and night. Each man was always new, and she forgot him in ten minutes.

Just Rocks

In another hall in the same building, a guy named Harry always entertained us. This guy was obsessed with rocks. We always knew where Harry had been as there were little rock piles all over the building. I am pretty sure he was building something pretty profound in his mind. We would even find rocks in his drawers, and around his room. He was never bored of rocks thank goodness. How is it possible you can be totally happy with rocks, but thank goodness it *is* possible. This particular home always had something interesting happening when I visited.

It is time for some Lexus

The last person who stands out there to me was a woman named Irene. She clearly had made good money in her life and liked to still dress in hats daily. She drove fancy cars and actually would frequently talk about owning a Lexus. The other thing she really liked was scotch. This facility actually kept a nice bottle of scotch for her in the office. I would always be sitting with the facility nurse, Yselaine, when she would come in the office asking for her Lexus. "Is it time for Lexus, do you know where I can find some Lexus." Well Irene was looking for her scotch, which she called Lexus. I was always shocked when Yselaine would give her a hit of scotch. I asked her what she did after the third or fourth time she came for a bit of Lexus. This woman could knock a few down easily. Yselaine ran through the several lies she used to keep her out of the bottle. Despite the notice that it was last call, Irene was always so happy and laughing, I always thought if I had dementia, this is who I would want to be like. Well, this is not completely true, I would be asking for a keg.

The Panera Cookie

The last story I call the Panera cookie story. It's a story about a guy named Max, seen for depression. I have known him quite a while as well. He lost his wife and has not been the same since then. I always find him the same, never real happy and not really sad. He is just there. He had started crying again and it raised the nurse's concern. I asked him if he was feeling depressed. He let me know he missed his family and he otherwise was fine. He asked for a cookie, and all we had is boring graham crackers. I had just gotten the most awesome chocolate chip cookie from Panera. It was sitting in my pocket calling my name. I love my chocolate, but I knew this guy probably had not had cookie that good in while. I asked the nurse if he was diabetic, and that's when she saw the cookie as well. He was in his late 80s, sad, and wanted a cookie. I sat and thought about how much insulin he would need later if I gave in. I asked the nurse, "Should I?" She said, "Yes, go ahead." It was worth the smile he gave, eyes big on the cookie. A little minute of sheer pleasure. I saw him the next week alive and well, and I was feeling relieved he did not die of diabetic coma.

I could tell hundreds of stories about what I have seen in nursing homes. I think the bottom line is finding someone's Panera cookie. It represents what that person loves and needs to have some quality of life. For Harry was a rock, Irene wanted her Lexus, and Max needed his cookie. All throughout life, you think about what you have to "get" to make you happy. Is it going to be a pool, a vacation, or a new home? Then you go work in a nursing home for years, and your perspective of what makes you happy changes. You think that being able to eat on our own, to walk, and maybe even to run are the most important things you will ever have. You realize that to have someone sitting in your room to say hello—anyone—can be one of the biggest part of your day. Learning to be happy with very little is an accomplishment that seems rare nowadays. If you ever have a chance to go to a nursing home, do it. It will always remind you of how much you have and how much you could lose. On my worst days when I feel sorriest for myself, my little love nuggets remind me of how much I really have. Learning to be grateful is one our biggest life lessons.

This is the end of the book, I discussed a lot of issues for you to consider. We are all in this aging process together and I hope we can all work together. The doctors, nurses, residents and families to all be on the same page would be nirvana. If I had to end on one thought, it would not be one you have never heard before, just one that needs to be spoken over and over again. Live each day as if it could be your last, whether you are sick or well, with dementia or without, no matter where your body is at the moment. No one is promised tomorrow on this earth.

About the Author

KAREN SEVERSON, M.D., was raised near the University of Connecticut in Storrs, famously known for cow tipping during down times. She grew up with her mother, father, and four siblings. They all played sports and had some wicked good snowball fights. She went to Ithaca College to become a Physical Education teacher. After hating that major and switching to a Biology nerd, Dr. Severson went into medical school on advice from a Chemistry teacher. He said she had a good memory! Dr. Severson's world changed after her mother developed breast cancer and died in medical school at the University of Connecticut. She really was impacted by her death and suffering and swore it would not be in vain. Dr. Severson later went to Brown University to complete her Psychiatry Residency training. She decided early she wanted to help the elderly and spent even more time completing a Fellowship in Geriatric Psychiatry at Albert Einstein College of Medicine in New York. The next 20 years of her life was spent treating elderly in hospitals and nursing homes. Dr. Severson never stopped thinking about how to make the lives of people suffering from terminal illness better. She had to write this book before she herself died.

Dr. Severson is married to an amazing wife with three daughters and she makes sure to teach them girl power daily. She still plays flag football, tae kwon do, and soccer, but needs to tone it down. She keeps breaking bones! Dr. Severson works more in the addiction field now, wanting to try to save young lives. One day she will retire in that Woodstock Nursing home, always trying to laugh and have a good time.